A LITTLE BIT

OF

AYURVEDA

A LITTLE BIT
OF
AYURVEDA

AN INTRODUCTION TO
AYURVEDIC MEDICINE

BY DEACON CARPENTER

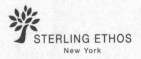

STERLING ETHOS
New York

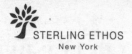

STERLING ETHOS
New York

An Imprint of Sterling Publishing
1166 Avenue of the Americas
New York, NY 10036

ISBN 978-1-4549-3641-1

Distributed in Canada by Sterling Publishing Co., Inc.
c/o Canadian Manda Group, 664 Annette Street
Toronto, Ontario M6S 2C8, Canada
Distributed in the United Kingdom by GMC Distribution Services
Castle Place, 166 High Street, Lewes, East Sussex BN7 1XU, England
Distributed in Australia by NewSouth Books
University of New South Wales, Sydney, NSW 2052, Australia

For information about custom editions, special sales, and premium and corporate purchases, please contact
Sterling Special Sales at 800-805-5489 or specialsales@sterlingpublishing.com.

Manufactured in Canada

2 4 6 8 10 9 7 5 3 1

sterlingpublishing.com

Cover design by Elizabeth Mihaltse Lindy
Interior design by Gina Bonanno

Illustrations by Marina Demidova *(kapha mandala)*/Shutterstock.com satit_srihin/Shutterstock.com (border)

CONTENTS

INTRODUCTION

How to Use This Book

More and more, we are learning that stress, poor diet, and an inactive lifestyle are major contributing factors to a rapidly increasing number of lifestyle diseases (obesity, diabetes, heart disease, high blood pressure, and depression) in our busy and constantly connected world. It as if we've forgotten some basic programming, like eating clean, exercising, and meditating—simple tools for disease prevention that we can use in our daily lives. We are shocked when we visit our doctor and learn that we have been diagnosed with a lifestyle disease, even though our lifestyles largely reflect choices that create stress, exhaustion, and a lack of connection with our body.

Understanding how our mind and bodily functions react to stress, and understanding how disease and illness are linked to diet, lifestyle, and the reduction of stress, are the foundations of Ayurveda. This ancient and complex medical system encompasses specific guidelines that are designed to prevent disease and illness and encourage us to live more healthy and balanced lives in accordance with the ebb and flow of nature. Ayurveda provides us with clear guidelines on how to live our lives with the innate understanding of our unique mind and body types (called *doshas*) and how to keep them balanced through the journey of life. In this book, you will learn that the principles of Ayurveda are relatively easy to comprehend, start to understand your own unique mind and body type, and see how this 5,000-year-old system is still highly relevant in modern society today.

First and foremost, this book is not to be used to diagnose or replace any medical or pharmaceutical protocols you have already been prescribed by your doctor. It is to be used to start the conversation of change from disease management to disease prevention and, in some cases, treatment. *A Little Bit of Ayurveda* will help you understand the different body/mind types, (doshas), as well as understand how untreated stress keeps us in the cycle of disease. It will help you learn effective rituals and remedies specific to your unique body/mind type and how to stay healthy through the cycle of the seasons and throughout the cycle of your life.

For many health seekers who are looking to Ayurveda or any alternative or CAM (complementary and alternative medicine) therapy for a "magic pill" or "magic treatment" solution, I have some unfortunate news: *there is no magic pill*—if there were such a pill or treatment, we would all be taking it. Ayurveda is truly personalized medicine that requires an individualized approach for each of us. Even if your diagnosis is similar to many other people's, your physiology and pathology (path to disease) are unique to you. By that, I mean that if you have a room of twenty people who have been diagnosed with breast cancer, there will be twenty unique physiologies and pathologies in the room.

The treatment for this disease may be similar, but each case is unique to the individual and will be different based on the patient's lifestyle, diet, and willingness to undergo the treatment.

We are all on our own health journey, and what may work wonders for one person may not be the best fit for another.

Ayurveda helps guide us to an understanding of the uniqueness of our own body and how to keep it healthy and disease free. Ayurveda has a strong focus on *measurable* and *long-term* results because of its emphasis on getting to the root of the disease or imbalance, rather than simply managing the symptoms of the disease.

We really only truly learn when we filter our knowledge through our own experiences. As this book starts to unfold, I invite you to look at the knowledge of Ayurveda as more of a framework than a collection of hard and fast rules for how to balance your mind and body. Approaching Ayurveda as a framework of knowledge allows more room for you to tailor it to your own body and lifestyle.

My journey to understanding started in 1988, shortly after I moved to the United States from the United Kingdom. I was pushing 275 lbs., with terrible cases of eczema and asthma. In the first year of living in the US, I gained an additional 60 lbs. I was tipping the scales at 330 lbs., and it was my friend Virginia (who I affectionately call my stepmother) who took me to my first yoga retreat and introduced me to Ayurveda. Just by changing my diet and lifestyle, incorporating yoga, and starting meditation (I practice Transcendental Meditation), I was able to lose half my body weight (I was 160 lbs. at my lowest), and my symptoms of eczema and asthma cleared up. I was hooked, and I knew at some point in my life, I would help people like me get well through this system.

Naturally, my journey is unique, as it will be for you. It's my intention that *A Little Bit of Ayurveda* will help you better understand what may seem to be a rather complex system that, until recently, was often relegated to the New Age movement. In reality, Ayurveda is fairly simple once you understand its principles along with your unique constitution and how to apply the knowledge of prevention. Consider this book as somewhat of a "user's manual" for your body.

It's also my intention for this book to help bridge the gap between Ayurveda and modern medicines, as we cannot have one without the other.

❖ 1 ❖

5,000 YEARS OF KNOWLEDGE ON HEALTH AND WELL-BEING

SOMETIMES KNOWN AS THE "GRANDPARENT" OF modern medicine, Ayurveda was created and codified in India more than 5,000 years ago. It is frequently referred to as "the sister philosophy" of yoga and is different in its approach from the modern medical model because its focus is on the whole patient (mental/physical/emotional) and the patient's unique bodily constitution, rather than just examining and managing the imbalance or disease the patient is experiencing.

In a nutshell, Ayurveda is personalized medicine.

The root of Ayurveda comes from the hymns (*Slokas*) of the *Upanishads*—sacred scriptures of Hinduism that were cognized and written by *rishi* (sages). Although part of a much bigger body of knowledge, it is thought that Ayurveda was born in the Indus Valley of North West India (now known as Pakistan) as part of the Vedanta philosophy of Hinduism.[1]

Within the scriptures of the Upanishads are the four Vedas (knowledge bases): the *Rig Veda*, the *Yajurveda*, the *Samavada*, and the *Atharvedaveda*. Each of the Vedas contain "applied sciences," or concepts for living in accordance with nature known as *Upavedas*. Upavedas include applied sciences such as government, architecture, art and music, and medicine.

Ayurveda comes from the *Rig Veda* and focuses on keeping the mind and body healthy and balanced through diet, lifestyle, and detoxification programs to prevent illness and treat disease. Ayurveda is not passive; it requires us to be proactive in managing our stress, eating seasonally and moderately, staying active, and engaging in self-care.

DEFINING AYURVEDA

The word Ayurveda is a combination of two words: Ayur (Ayus) meaning "life" and Veda (Ved), meaning "knowledge." Translated, Ayurveda means "knowledge of life" and, most specifically, knowledge of you and how to understand your own mind and body type, stress triggers, and what to do when you get sick. Ayurveda provides a vast body of knowledge on the specific needs of our body and mind. The notion of "self-referral" guides us to sustained and balanced health and helps prevent diseases.

The term *self-referral* is commonly used to describe a person's understanding or point of reference to their own mind and body type and if an experience will bring them into or take them out of balance. For example, you may love the summer, but you know that if you don't wear sunscreen and you're out in the sun for more than ten minutes, you're guaranteed to burn. This is because your particular body type is more sensitive to the sun than others. Ayurveda gives us the knowledge of the traits of our unique mind and body type (dosha) and reminds us how important it is to refer back to that knowledge to prevent disease and stay balanced.

Ayurveda has two main goals:

1. To preserve the health of the healthy—keeping you balanced throughout the journey of your life.
2. To eradicate disease and imbalances in the sick—focusing on reversing the disease process and removing toxins and pathogens from the body to "cure" the physiology of disease.

Ayurveda has influenced many other medical systems, including Traditional Chinese Medicine, Greek and Islamic medicine, and even modern medicine. Ayurveda was the first system to categorize medicine into eight branches: internal medicine, surgery, pediatrics, psychology, ENT (ear, nose, and throat), toxicology, gerontology, and fertility.[2] In more recent history, Ayurveda has been classified as a complementary and alternative medicine (CAM) to modern medicine.[3]

However, more and more health-care providers are finding that their patients and clients are experiencing sustainable results when it comes to their overall health and well-being by incorporating techniques such as stress reduction (like meditation or breathing exercises), more moderate and "cleaner" diets (reducing processed foods and eating more seasonally), movement programs (like yoga), and lifestyle edits such as getting better sleep, being more active, and being part of a community.

These cues are essentially the Ayurvedic approach to living, and in my ten years of experience, I've seen my clients and patients experience a reduction in pharmaceutical use (in partnership with their Western doctors), a reduction in gastrointestinal inflammation (GERD, diverticulitis, IBS, and others), a reduction in lifestyle diseases (obesity, high blood pressure, type II diabetes) and chronic pain, and in some cases a reduction in anxiety and depression.

With Ayurveda, prevention is the name of the game. Although Ayurveda does provide purgative protocols for "curing" chronic and long-term disease (called Panchakarma—Ayurveda's version of surgery), it cannot be used allopathically. By that, I mean Ayurveda is more effective when used preventively. Modern medicine provides us with emergency care, intervention, and management of disease when we are in urgent need of it. Ayurveda provides us with disease prevention by identifying what may be causing us ill health before it gets worse.

I believe that there is a place for Ayurveda (and any other integrative or CAM therapies) to work in harmony with modern medicine. All paths to health!

Remember that your journey to balanced health is exactly that—*your* journey. Your body is as unique as you are. Although I've provided you with some guidelines about each of the Ayurvedic mind and body types, it is with the intention that you will research and discover more about your unique health and well-being needs through Ayurveda and yoga.

I encourage you to avoid the "all or nothing" approach as you start seeking balance and changing your habits. Start where you feel most comfortable, making changes that are easy for you, and over time begin to include better habits. Small victories lead to sustainable results.

❖ 2 ❖

MODERN USE
AND PRACTICAL
APPLICATION OF
AYURVEDA

I WOULD LIKE TO PRESENT YOU WITH A RATHER simple saying that one of my early teachers always used, that stuck with me when I started my journey into Ayurvedic medicine in my late teens: *"Water the root to enjoy the fruit."* This notion resonated with me so deeply, it continues to be my mantra in my clinical practice as I work with my clients; the root of the problem is where we start—not at the leaf, flower, or fruit.

In Ayurveda, when a person is not well, we don't look at a skin rash, bad temper, or acid reflux in treatment; these are symptoms of the cause. Instead, we learn what sort of foods that person is consuming, what his stress levels look like, if he is sleeping well, and if he is using substances (food, alcohol, recreational or pharmaceutical drugs) to cope with stress. Once we can understand the root cause of the problem, we can start to solve it and thereby reduce the skin rash, bad temper, acid reflux, or any other issue. Otherwise, all we are doing is managing the patient's symptoms.

In modern medicine, however, we don't typically start at the root of our problem; rather, we typically seek medications and treatments that often simply mask or reduce the symptoms of our problem. This allows us to cope and just "get on" with our busy lives, rather than fix the problem at the root. We are too busy to get sick!

THE STRESS FACTOR IN GETTING SICK

Unless we are gravely ill or going through a major health crisis, we prefer to "power through" an illness and regard it as an inconvenience, rather than a chance to rest and truly get better. It's only when we encounter a true health crisis (stroke, heart attack, or something else) that we start to reconsider our overall well-being, and even then, we tend to rely more heavily on the prescribed protocols from conventional doctors, rather than really and truly changing our lifestyle habits and evolving our diet. It's almost as if we have been made redundant and do not need to be an active participant in understanding our body as it relates to taking care of our own health and well-being.

The challenge with not being thoughtful about treating the root of illness is that we don't know how the illness started in the first place. We aren't tuned in to the little warnings and notifications our body may be sending us: a skin rash, tension headaches, loose bowels, anxiety, and others. We often don't understand how our own mind and body work together in order to be effective at preventing disease—instead, we are pushed into a reactive state of mind when we get sick, and I mean REALLY sick. If we only knew how to read the subtle warning signs as we are about to get sick, we could be more proactive. We need to find our "check engine" light, so to speak.

In my experience as an Ayurvedic specialist, stress reduction and management are directly linked to our overall state of health, but many of us are too busy with work to think about reducing our stress.

Even though not regulated by federal law, most workers in the US earn two weeks' vacation time every year.[4] These precious two weeks are put in place so that we can take paid time off from work in order to recharge our batteries, gain perspective on our direction in life, and reduce the accumulated stress from working long and hard. Ironically, this time off work is intended to make us more productive and happy as employees.

Of course, unplugging from work stress in a highly competitive job market isn't always possible or acceptable—especially the farther your career takes you; and because we are always connected to work through a company laptop or mobile device, there is an unspoken expectation of always being "on."

In my seventeen years' experience climbing the corporate ladder in the US, much of this control comes from fear regarding job security. We feel as if we MUST be involved in a project at every step so that we are an integral part of it and, therefore, invaluable to the company and "unsackable." It's as if some of us are pathologically unable to take the time off for fear of losing our job.

CAREER FEAR

Fear makes us work longer hours, causing us to be unable to reduce our stress, leading to more sickness and not taking sick days.

When I was working for a global advertising agency in New York, our client was a large technology company based in the San Francisco Bay Area. I was responsible for managing a large international team, which meant multiple time zones, cultures, and languages, as well as highly demanding clients and completely unreasonable deadlines. I was working up to 100 hours per week and traveling all over the world, making sure my team in New York did their job properly.

Even though it wasn't mandated at work, it was quietly expected that we were to be on call twenty-four hours per day. A missed email could lead to a global fire, and I would be one of the ones to face the blame.

It was during a challenging project with unrealistic deadlines that the flu was going around our office. It started with one of the account managers and quickly spread to the creative team, then the production team, and finally my team. Generally, when a person has the flu, rest is required with lots of fluids; but we *couldn't* rest. We were already grossly understaffed, and many of us were doing the job of three employees. What happened was pretty remarkable: we would be sick for two to three weeks, feel better for a week, then get sick again. It was clearly stress that caused the flu to be as unrelenting as our projects. Stress affects our sleep, it affects our diet (we will consume more convenient/packaged foods), lifestyle, and relationships with others; it impacts our health negatively. [5]

This isn't the case in other parts of the world, however. In the UK, workers are legally entitled to 5.6 paid weeks off per year. That's twenty-eight paid vacation days to decompress from the job, and the clear message that it is a priority to take time off—it's the law! [6]

FEELING WELL THROUGH SELF-REFERRAL

In addition to stress reduction, the third and most important part of understanding how to prevent diseases is knowing what it means to feel well. Many of us in the West have never truly had the experience of what it feels like to feel good in our mind and in our body—we only aspire to feel as well as how we think others feel. We often focus on how we should be feeling, rather than how we could be feeling. Understanding our own sense of well-being is one of the foundational concepts of Ayurvedic medicine and is called self-referral.

The knowledge of our own self-referral and a true understanding of what being well feels like helps us pay attention to the first signs of illness so that we can prevent it from progressing; plus it gives us the ability to prevent similar stressful situations in the future.

If we don't understand the natural state and tendencies of our unique mind and body type, if we don't understand the journey of disease in our own body, being able to find relief or a cure will be difficult and will result in more chronic illness over time.

HOW AYURVEDA WORKS

The knowledge of Ayurveda provides us with something like a user's manual for our physiology and psychology, based on our unique mind and body combination (dosha). When it comes to getting sick (or experiencing an imbalance, as it's known in Ayurveda), knowledge of self provides us with a solid baseline of health, depending on our unique constitution, or "doshic type." Understanding the nature and quality of our state of homeostasis, or balance, helps us to understand what imbalances we are prone to, how to spot an imbalance before it starts, and what to do when we go out of balance, as well as how to prevent the imbalance from going farther.

Having the knowledge and wisdom of how our individual mind/body type functions and fluctuates gives us a much deeper understanding of how to get back to our roots of health and balance. Ayurveda examines the quality of our diet, the level of activity in our lifestyle, and our stress level. Ayurveda employs treatments such as corrective diet, meditation, yoga asana, breathing exercises, and herbal protocols to help bring the body back into balance.

To be clear, I'm NOT against modern medicine at all. It is an absolutely indispensable and necessary technology for disease intervention and emergency treatment. What I am suggesting, however, is that lifestyle diseases such as high blood pressure, type II diabetes, obesity, and in some cases, depression can actually be greatly mitigated, if not cured, with the combination of modern medicine and Ayurvedic protocols.

THE DOCTOR AS TEACHER AND STUDENT

The traditional name given to Ayurvedic practitioners is Vaidya. The term Vaidya not only means doctor but also teacher. This is a very important distinction between modern medicine and Ayurveda, as your vaidya won't just be treating your imbalances when you're sick but also teaching you how to stay balanced in your daily life by teaching you about your unique mind/body type (dosha), which allows you to hone your ability to have self-referral.

Vaidyas can only teach what they were taught through their own experience. As they don't live in your body, they don't know what kind of stress triggers you have and what mechanisms you use when coping with stress (eating, using substances, or others). Educating you on how to prevent illness and imbalance as they relate to your unique constitution is part of the journey back to balance. Ayurveda requires you to be an active participant in your health and well-being, and vaidyas facilitate that process.

AYURVEDA'S RELATIONSHIP TO YOGA

In many circles in the West, Ayurveda is most commonly referred to as a "sister" philosophy of yoga. However, I've always felt that this statement makes Ayurveda less important than it really is. As you investigate the relationship between Ayurveda and yoga, you will discover that Ayurveda and yoga share a much more integral and symbiotic relationship with each other. In fact, I would venture to say that if you aren't practicing Ayurveda with yoga, you're not getting the full benefit of your practice.

In Ayurveda, knowledge is merely theory without experience; we need experience to truly understand how to interact with and apply the knowledge we've learned. We connect the dots of the knowledge through our personal experience. Ayurveda is the knowledge of how to live life according to the flow of nature. This covers the understanding of our unique constitution, how our body reacts to seasonal changes, how we mitigate and cope with stress, how to be mindful and practice self-care when it is necessary, and how to know when to walk away from certain situations that can cause imbalance.

Yoga is how we experience the knowledge through our unique journey: knowing how we react to certain situations and stress, knowing what to do when we are feeling under the weather, and observing the experience of our unique physiology and psychology throughout our lives. We can't have the experience (yoga) without the knowledge (Ayurveda), and vice versa.

For example, when we were toddlers, we bumped into everything as we learned to move. Our parents cautiously watched over us, making sure that we didn't harm ourselves. We didn't completely understand how items in the house could cause us pain without the experience of hurting ourselves by colliding with these items.

We don't fully understand the concept of "hot" until we encounter something hot to the touch for the first time and we feel the heat and fear of that experience. Our parents try to communicate their knowledge and experience of "hot" to our developing minds by yelling the word, hoping that it will, in some way, prevent us from touching the hot item. However, the only way we can understand that HOT hurt us is by touching a hot item and burning ourselves.

Ayurveda is the knowledge of "hot" our parents are attempting to teach us. Yoga is the experience of burning ourselves. We've been able to connect the knowledge of "hot" with the experience of "burn." Experience gives us a point of reference. It helps us determine our tolerance for pain, sadness, anger, or serenity. This is how we experience life on the most fundamental level.

If you'd rather understand the interaction in a way that doesn't involve physical pain, consider how to bake a cake. When you think about baking a cake, you first think about what sort of flavors and textures you desire, what you need in order to produce it. The ingredients, the utensils, and the oven temperature. The knowledge of why you mix dry ingredients together with wet ingredients, why you cream butter and sugar together, and why you whip egg whites prior to folding them into your batter. That knowledge represents Ayurveda.

Implementing that knowledge with action represents yoga—measuring out exactly two cups of flour, preheating the oven to 350°F, and gently folding in those fluffy egg whites into the batter. That is the yoga of making a cake. The movements and actions executed with intention.

❈ 3 ❈

FIVE ELEMENTS, THREE DOSHAS, AND THEIR QUALITIES

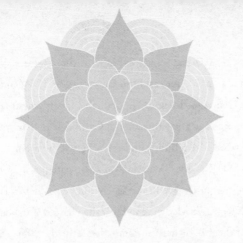

V ERY ENCOURAGINGLY, MORE AND MORE modern medical doctors in the US are touting the benefits of preventive care through complementary alternative medicine (CAM).[7] In fact, the practice of Functional Medicine, which is an up-and-coming specialty for Western doctors and has the same approach to disease as Ayurveda, treats the root cause, not the symptoms.[8] As many people are living with "lifestyle diseases" like type 2 diabetes, high blood pressure, obesity, and inflammatory digestive diseases, there is a much larger need for us to be active participants in our own health care and well-being. In fact, a 2017 study by the Center for disease control (CDC) claimed that of the $3.3 trillion in US health-care expenditures, 90 percent of these expenditures involved patients with chronic lifestyle diseases.[9]

Conventional doctors are being trained in complementary alternative medical therapies now more than ever before. Many institutions include programs for alternative medicine, such as the

University of Arizona, which is home to the Andrew Weil Center for Integrative Medicine, and the University of Maryland School of Medicine Center for Integrative Medicine. Health organizations like Johns Hopkins and the University of California at San Francisco not only embrace CIM (clinical and investigative medicine) and CAM therapies but also offer Ayurveda to their patients. In Canada, the Canadian Integrative Medical Association helps doctors find fellowships in Integrative Medicine in both the US and Canada.

Many health insurance companies already offer coverage for acupuncture, meditation, and medical massage. Many companies in the US offer Flexible Spending or Health Savings accounts that can cover these therapies and can allow employees to save thousands of dollars tax-free per year and spend the money on preventive care. Although these programs are not perfect, they are progress, and the conversation is changing toward prevention.

ELEMENTS, DOSHAS, AND THE NATURE OF AYURVEDA

There are two fundamental concepts in Ayurveda: the five-element theory (pancha mahabuthas) and the three-energies model (tri dosha).

The Ayurvedic body of knowledge defines the five elements as space, air, fire, water, and earth. There are two rules we accept in Ayurveda when looking at the five-element theory: The first is that in order to understand how each of the five elements exists and operates in nature, we must understand their qualities. The second is that this theory is applied to all matter, both organic and inorganic, in the *entire* universe, ranging from the most expansive areas of space right down to the smallest atom on Earth. Everything that manifests (or has the potential to manifest) is associated with one or more of the five elements.

More importantly, when the five-element theory is applied to our own mind and body, we can start to define the governing principles of each of the five elements as they relate to our unique body and mind combination and understand how they can influence our physical and emotional health when our health is in or out of balance.

When we look at the five elements we must also look at their innate qualities, which describe how they function in nature and in the mind and body. There are twenty qualities (gunas) related to the five elements, and each of the five elements has up to nine qualities each!

The twenty qualities are heavy, dull, cold, oily, smooth, dense, hard, static, subtle, cloudy, light, sharp, hot, dry, rough, liquid, soft, mobile, gross, and clear.

FIVE-ELEMENT THEORY:
PANCHA MAHABUTHAS

SPACE (*Akasha*) is the idea of connectedness and expansiveness. Space exists between things, and it also imperceptibly connects everything together. Space is so subtle that we cannot perceive it with our senses, although we are conscious that it exists. It is the subtlest form of matter and is the fabric that all creation is built from. In the body, space represents the cavities, or empty spaces, that exist. In the mind, space represents our connected consciousness.

The qualities of space are cold, dry, light, subtle, flowing, sharp, and clear.

AIR *(Vayu)* is the idea of motion. Whatever moves in nature is propelled by air. Wind is the physical representation of air, and air is the force behind all motion. It is the force that moves a butterfly or hummingbird, an airplane or a person's arm. Air is not just oxygen—it governs all movement in the body and in the universe. In the body, air governs the movement of the nerve impulses, the breath, the ability to speak, the movement of digestion and elimination through the body, and the movement of limbs. In the mind, air governs thought.

The qualities of air are cold, dry, light, subtle, flowing, sharp, hard, rough, and clear.

FIRE *(Tejas)* is the idea of light, heat, and transformation. It is obvious that fire is hot and that it gives off both heat and light. Its transformative property is seen in its power to change a solid into a liquid. Fire represents the force of our evolution, converting who we are into who we are becoming. Fire creates the heat of fevers, illuminates truth, and dispels ignorance. In the body, fire governs digestion and metabolism. In the mind it governs perception and discernment.

The qualities of fire are hot, dry, light, subtle, flowing, sharp, hard, rough, and clear.

WATER *(Apas)* is the idea of flow and liquidity. Water represents the liquid form of matter. It has no inherent motion of its own but flows along the path of least resistance. Water not only represents water in the body, but all liquids including liquid metals, oils, and fluids. In the body, water represents fluidity. In the mind, it represents loving and compassionate emotions.

The qualities of water are cold, moist, heavy, gross, static, dull, soft, smooth, and cloudy.

EARTH *(Prithivi)* is the idea of stability. Wood, metal, plastic, a blade of grass, and other matter are all comprised of the idea of solidity. Each example simply represents the solid form of matter and the principle that stability is provided in the grossest form. In the body, earth represents physical structure, cohesion, and growth. In the mind, it represents mental stability.

The qualities of earth are moist, dry, heavy, gross, dense, static, dull, hard, rough, and cloudy.

The guidelines when understanding the qualities (*gunas*) of the elements are that like will increase like, hot will increase hot, cold will increase cold, gross will increase gross, and so on. With that in mind, when we are thinking about treating an imbalance or bringing mind and body back into balance, we typically don't fight fire with fire; we fight fire with water or earth. We also don't look at increasing one element to decrease another. That just makes it harder to come back to balance, and then we have two elements to work on.

THE THREE ENERGIES: TRI DOSHA MODEL

Translated literally, the word *dosha* means, "that which can become faulty, cause imbalance, or go wrong." The definition alone clues us in to the fact that balancing our dosha is an ongoing journey and, for some of us, can feel like a bit of a chore. Ayurveda's focus is squarely on understanding our own coping tendencies (samskaras) when we encounter stress and how to mitigate and prevent health imbalances.

Each of the three doshas is comprised of a combination of the five elements (space, air, fire, water, and earth). By combining the five elements into the three doshas, we can understand much more clearly how the elements and their qualities interact to influence our mind and body.

Vata: Space and Air

The qualities of Vata (space and air) are dry, light, cold, mobile, clear, rough, hard, and subtle. Vata is responsible for movement, transportation, and communication.

Expansive and mobile are the traits of Vata. The element of space is vast and expansive, and the element of air governs movement. Because of this, Vata is the only dosha of the three that is mobile; the other two doshas are static. Air allows the fire element to burn, the water element to flow, and the earth element to solidify. Vata is the facilitator, allowing the doshas to be dynamic.

The combination of space and air is vast and variable and great for big ideas but also conveys Vata's fundamental qualities of mobility and light and perhaps being a little too "out there."

Pitta: Fire and Water

The qualities of Pitta (fire and water) are oily, light, hot, sharp, mobile, and liquid. Pitta is responsible for digestion, transformation, and discernment.

Combustible and transformative are the traits of Pitta. The water element in Pitta is more oily in nature and generally refers to the gastric juices in the digestive system and their ability to transform food into energy and tissues. The fire element in Pitta ignites the flame in our digestion, and in combination with the gastric juices, allows us to have a healthy metabolism.

Oil and fire are a volatile mix, which is great for metabolism but this also speaks to the fundamental qualities of being hot and sharp and perhaps being a little hotheaded.

Kapha: Water and Earth

The qualities of Kapha (water and earth) are dull, oily, heavy, cold, slow, smooth, dense, cloudy, and soft. Kapha is responsible for structure, lubrication, and growth.

Solid and grounded are the traits of Kapha. The water element protects our joints and the lining of body organs, and the earth element provides growth and structure to our body.

Mixing water with earth gives you mud, which is important for building but also indicates Kapha's fundamental quality of being sticky and dense and perhaps being "stuck in the mud."

STATE OF BALANCE VERSUS STATE OF IMBALANCE: PRAKRUTI AND VIKRUTI

Ayurvedic principles use the concepts of the three doshas to identify the qualities of the constitution of a person (prakruti) as well as the qualities of that person's imbalance (vikruti).

Your prakruti is the concept of mind/body constitution and is determined at the time of conception. Your prakruti is based on family genetics, heritage, and the quality of your parents' reproductive organs. Your prakruti will not change over the course of your life; if you were born a Vata type, you will always be a Vata type.

Vikruti, however, is the concept of the constant state of change and balance in your mind and body and does change over time. Essentially, vikruti is the intelligence of your body when you are stressed, not eating properly, not getting good-quality sleep, and generally not taking care of yourself. Vikruti is smarter than you are—it knows your body type and where you are more prone to get sick. If you are Pitta and aren't taking care of yourself, your vikruti will cause a Pitta-genic imbalance in your body. It might be mild at first, but the more you justify your behavior to "cope" and do not balance your body, the worse the symptoms will get and the harder the imbalance will be to resolve.

In addition to not tending to our state of well-being when we are stressed, other factors that cause our vikruti to become imbalanced are the change of seasons (for example, summer to fall), change in age, and change in routines and lifestyles.

OVERVIEW OF THE THREE DOSHAS

Each of the three doshas has very specific physical and emotional traits associated with it due to the qualities of their elements. Even though these are fairly general observations about each of them, they may accurately resonate with you based on your own body type.

Vata

THE ECTOMORPH :: THE BUTTERFLY ::
THE ESOTERIC ARTIST AND THE SOCIALITE

Vatas tend to be vibrant, generally, and have an intoxicating excitement for life.

Being light in nature, their usually positive outlook translates to an energetic expression that is contagious to their friends. They are light of heart, are quick to speak, and typically have their head in the clouds, both figuratively and literally!

However, as Vata is a combination of space and air, they can sometimes become spacey and erratic with their work, relationships, and approach to life in general—especially when they have to commit to a plan, deadline, or deliverable of any kind. Mixing the expansiveness of space and the unpredictability of air can cause Vata to be ungrounded and unsure of themselves. This variability can cause anxiety, which in some cases can lead to depression.

The Vata personality is best described as that of a butterfly—able to move with the wind, flutter quickly about, and change direction rapidly and often. People with a Vata personality have many interests and do not travel down one path for too long, as they tend to get distracted very easily. Vatas are bubbly when things are grounded, but when that delicate balance is upset, they tend toward fear and anxiety, and can become overwhelmed quickly. Think of a butterfly caught in a windstorm.

When out of balance due to being ungrounded and pulled in many different directions (sometimes by their own restless minds) Vatas tend to be all over the place. They often struggle when forced to make life-changing decisions. They can vacillate between feeling that the choice they made was absolutely the right one and worrying for days at a time that it wasn't.

In the physical body, Vata represents MOVEMENT (heart rate, respiratory system, physical movement), TRANSPORTATION (blood circulation, movement of the digestive system), ELIMINATION/removal of waste from the body (urine, feces, and sweat), and COMMUNICATION (the ability to think and speak). When Vata goes out of balance in the body, people experience symptoms like atrial fibrillation and hyperventilation (MOVEMENT). Cold extremities, gas, and bloating can occur (TRANSPORTATION). Dry stools and scant urination can occur (ELIMINATION). Speech may become impaired or too fast and the thought process can become erratic (COMMUNICATION).

PHYSICAL TRAITS OF VATA

❋ High forehead

❋ Receding chin

❋ Narrow shoulders and hips

❋ Narrow chest and abdomen

❋ Thin arms and legs

❋ Little subcutaneous fat

EMOTIONAL TRAITS OF VATA

❋ Inspirational

❋ Creative

❋ Anxiety prone

❋ Worrying

ADJECTIVES FOR VATA

❋ Positive: Creative, inspired, energetic, enthusiastic, fun, lighthearted

❋ Neutral: Fast, sensitive

❋ Challenging: Indecisive, unpredictable, scattered, flighty, spacey, moody, superficial

ORGANS AND SYSTEMS ASSOCIATED WITH VATA

❋ Brain: Frontal lobe—abstract thinking, motor functions, expressive language, regulator of emotions

❋ Temporal lobe—speech, auditory processing, emotions, and behavior

❋ Heart: Rhythm and frequency of heartbeat

❋ Lungs: Air and the drawing in of oxygen

❋ Colon: Defecation

❋ Bladder: Urination

❋ Bone marrow and nervous system: Efferent nerve impulses

PITTA :: THE MESOMORPH :: THE BULL :: THE NATURAL BORN LEADER AND THE DYNAMIC VISIONARY

Pittas generally tend to be warm and friendly to their friends and fierce opponents of their enemies (and "frenemies"). Being hot in nature, Pittas are strong-willed and dynamic leaders with passion and vision who can motivate others to see the Pitta vision and rally to the Pitta cause.

Pittas tend to speak clearly and with conviction and can convince others to be part of their project and vision. They can cut though arguments like a hot knife through butter and have very little time for those who put up a fight, get in the way, or deal in lengthy decision-making and bureaucracy. Pittas may be fantastic leaders and delegators, generally, but they sometimes let their competitive nature get in the way of things. Pittas aren't always the best at planning and project management, as they can be impetuous and hotheaded.

When Pittas are balanced and everything is going swimmingly, they are radiant and resolute. However, when things get hot and challenging, they can be recalcitrant and childish—attempting to assign blame (more commonly known as "blamestorming") and, in extreme cases, may even be slightly delusional and believe that they are being sabotaged or set up to fail.

When they set their sights on a target, no matter if it's a project, career, or relationship, Pittas charge straight ahead. This is the general approach of a Pitta and has been compared to a bull in a china shop—if you get in their way, you could get trampled, gored, or caught in their wake of carnage!

When imbalanced, Pitta personalities typically include qualities like being arrogant, highly competitive, overly brash, and easily angered. They will push for high standards and they are prone to overwork, which tends to lead to feeling overwhelmed and, eventually, to burnout. If they become emotionally imbalanced, their relationships can become challenging and even come to an end, as Pittas have the innate ability to burn bridges. Not all the time, of course, but it is always an option to them!

Pittas tend to be well organized and natural leaders but typically not too detail oriented, which can lead them to try to control certain situations even though they don't have all the facts. This comes from their desire to always be the leader in any and all situations by imposing their will.

The water quality for Pitta is more oily than that of Kapha, creating a more combustable mix of these elements. Pittas can use that combustion for innovation or annihilation—it all depends on their state of balance.

In the physical body, Pitta governs METABOLISM (of thoughts, food, and experiences), DIGESTION AND TRANSFORMATION (of food into tissues, of thoughts into opinions), and DISCERNMENT (of situations, lifestyle choices, and relationships).

When Pitta goes out of balance, symptoms of hyperacidity and heartburn can occur (METABOLISM). Diarrhea and inflammatory digestive disorders can occur (DIGESTION AND TRANSFORMATION). Addiction and poor lifestyle choices can occur (DISCERNMENT).

PHYSICAL TRAITS OF PITTA

- Medium build and height
- Broad shoulders
- Muscular arms and legs
- Narrow hips
- Some subcutaneous fat

EMOTIONAL TRAITS OF PITTA

- Aspirational
- Engaging
- Dynamic
- Critical
- Selfish

ADJECTIVES FOR PITTA

- Positive: Courageous, brave, focused, perceptive
- Neutral: Logical, organized, serious
- Challenging: Angry, jealous, envious, critical, sharp, judgmental

ORGANS AND SYSTEMS OF PITTA

- Skin: Color and temperature
- Eyes: Iris
- Liver: Act of metabolism
- Brain: Parietal lobe—sensory information, functions of taste, touch, smell, and temperature regulation
- Occipital lobe—Visual system, cognitive thought
- Blood: Color
- Spleen: Recycling of red blood cells
- Small intestine: Metabolism
- Endocrine system: Hormone regulation

KAPHA :: THE ENDOMORPH :: THE TURTLE :: THE PARENT, THE ROCK, AND THE CAREGIVER

Kaphas generally tend to be calm and methodical. They move, think, and react slowly and judiciously. Their steady disposition is not easily disturbed, and they tend to be loving and devoted individuals—characteristics that are reflective of the large amount of water in their constitutions.

Kaphas are the people in our lives we call our "rocks." They are the ones we seek out when we are having a rough day or need advice on a situation. They have a gentle and nurturing way about them, which makes it easy to confide in them.

Because of their denser and slower constitutions, Kaphas find it difficult to make changes, pick up new hobbies, or evolve their behavior patterns. Kaphas prefer to plod steadily along the path of life and like to fit into society rather than stand out.

Kaphas tend to have more of an analytical and conservative approach to projects, situations, and relationships. Kaphas lean toward accepting things the way they are so as to not rock the boat. They can also take the view of the world a little more pessimistically and with a glass-half-empty attitude. They are sometimes called the "stick in the mud" because of their attitude and lack of true motivation to change.

When Kaphas are out of balance, they become attached to and hold a feeling for a long time. They can become resentful in a relationship or situation and are notorious for holding a grudge. Kaphas can also be controlling when out of balance—not in the same sense as Pitta can in terms of a desire to impose their will but more in the sense of controlling a relationship or situation through conditional love and, in extreme cases, through blackmail.

In the physical body, Kapha governs **STRUCTURE** (bones of the body), **LUBRICATION** (waters and oils of the body), **COHESION** (ligaments and joints), and **GROWTH** (not just cysts, bumps, and lumps, but also growth from conception to young adulthood).

When Kapha goes out of balance, bones can develop spurs (**STRUCTURE**). Excess mucus and acne/oily skin can develop (**LUBRICATION**). Joints can be hypermobile and ligaments can be thick (**COHESION**). Cysts and other growths can appear (**GROWTH**).

PHYSICAL TRAITS OF KAPHA

❀ Pear-shaped body

❀ Large, rounded head

❀ Wide hips and shoulders

❀ Heavy or solid bones

❀ Many subcutaneous fat deposits

EMOTIONAL TRAITS OF KAPHA

❀ Kind and loving

❀ Mentoring

❀ Pessimistic

❀ Controlling

❀ Tendency to hold a grudge

ADJECTIVES FOR KAPHA

❀ Positive: Sweet, calm, loving, compassionate, nurturing, affectionate, gentle

❀ Neutral: Slow, steady, stoic, conservative, obedient

❀ Challenging: Stubborn, attached, controlling, rigid, complacent, uninspired

ORGANS AND SYSTEMS OF KAPHA

❀ Brain: Cerebellum—attention, rhythm, proprioception

❀ Cerebrospinal fluid: Protects the brain in the skull

❀ Joints: Cohesion, growth, and repair

❀ Mouth: Salivary glands and oral cavity lining

❀ Stomach: Stomach lining

❀ Pleural cavity: Lining of the lungs

❀ Pericardial cavity: Lining around the heart

❀ Lymphatic system: Regulation of the immune system

DIGESTION, METABOLISM, AND WASTE MANAGEMENT: THE ROOTS OF OUR HEALTH

THERE IS A PROVERB IN AYURVEDA: "WHEN DIET IS of poor quality, medicine is of no use. When diet is of good quality, medicine is of no need." This saying may have influenced Hippocrates (the father of modern medicine) when he said, "Let food be medicine and medicine be food."

In the Ayurvedic proverb, the word *diet* isn't referring to a plan to help encourage weight loss but to the quality of the foods we are consuming as well as the quality and strength of our digestive system in order to metabolize it effectively.

Chances are you've heard the expression "you are what you eat." In my experience of working with people and helping them to strengthen their digestive systems, the expression "you are what you can metabolize" is more succinct and accurate as it encompasses how your body can digest and metabolize food, assimilate nutrients, manage waste (sweat, urine, and feces—also called *mala*) and the residual and undigested food left behind in the digestive tract (called *ama*).

In Ayurveda, the digestive system is also referred to as the *inner disease pathway*, because it's essentially where disease pathology starts and, when our metabolism and digestion aren't functioning optimally, how disease can hitch a ride in the bloodstream as pathogenesis occurs from accumulated ama.

The concept of balance is simple. If we can keep imbalances in the digestive system and ama to a minimum, we can prevent disease from spreading throughout our body, and we will be able to stay balanced and disease free. The challenge, however, is that the little disturbances in the digestive system that we need to watch for to prevent an imbalance are subtle, and if we aren't trained in what to look for, we may miss a cue to prevent getting ill.

Ayurveda was conceived long before modern diagnostic machines (X-rays and CAT and PET scans) were invented. In Ayurveda, it is important to look at what is coming out of you—your waste products—to determine the type of imbalance or disease you are encountering.

AGNI: DIGESTIVE FIRE

Agni is the Sanskrit word for "fire" and indicates digestive or metabolic fire. The quality of your agni determines how your food is metabolized, how your body eliminates or holds onto waste, and how your immune system and every other system in the body stay healthy and function optimally—homeostasis.

There are four different types or "conditions" of agni, and they are directly related to the balance or imbalance of the doshas. They are normal, high, low, and variable.

Normal agni means that your digestive system is balanced, your food is being metabolized optimally, and your waste products (urine, feces, and sweat) are being produced and released optimally based on your dosha.

High agni is typically associated with people who have more of a Pitta constitution. When Pitta is imbalanced, the result could be inflammation and hyperacidity.

Low agni is typically associated with people who have more of a Kapha constitution. When Kapha is imbalanced, the result could be constant low-grade hunger and feeling heavy and sluggish.

Variable agni is typically associated with people who have more of a Vata constitution. When Vata is imbalanced, the result could be gas and distension.

MALA: WASTE PRODUCTS

Malas are the waste products of the body. They are urine, feces, and sweat. In Ayurveda, we look at the qualities of these waste products to determine if the body is metabolizing food properly or not (since we can't look inside you, we have to examine what's coming out of you).

There are four types of Mala qualities:

Normal mala means that your body is managing waste optimally, and everything is running optimally.

The waste products of people who are Vata are typically drier and less voluminous in nature, due to the combination of space and air. When experiencing an imbalance of Vata, symptoms generally include urine that is more scant or darker in color, bowel movements that are drier, harder to pass, and more infrequent (every 2–3 days), and scant sweat production.

The waste products of people who are predominantly Pitta are typically frequent and profuse, due to the combination of fire and water. When experiencing an imbalance of Pitta, symptoms generally include urgent urination that may feel hot, more frequent bowel movements (up to 5 per day) that are loose and more urgent, and profuse sweating that occurs more easily.

The waste products of those who are more Kapha, are typically regular and more voluminous, due to the combination of water and earth. When experiencing a Kapha imbalance, symptoms generally include excess urination, more voluminous and sticky bowel movements that may have mucus present, and reduced sweat.

AMA

Ama is the term for undigested food residue in the digestive tract.

Ama can form in the digestive tract over time due to low and variable agni (in Vata and Kapha types), poor-quality food consumption (packaged foods, highly processed foods, and so on), eating too rapidly or not chewing food properly, being distracted while eating, overeating, and having high stress levels.

If ama is not removed from the digestive system through diet and lifestyle, it will start to decay, causing diseases that may remain localized in the digestive system. If the situation is not resolved, the longer ama remains in the digestive system, the greater the chance pathogens will enter the bloodstream and find a new home elsewhere in your body.

THE DIGESTIVE PROCESS

Digestion starts in the mouth and includes the esophagus, stomach, small intestine, large intestine, and colon. The organs of digestion also include the liver, gallbladder, and pancreas.

Digestion starts in the mouth because the stomach doesn't have teeth. It's extremely important to chew your food—even smoothies. When you put food in your mouth and start to chew, the magic of digestion starts.

1. The brain sends a signal through the vagus nerve to increase production of saliva in the mouth. Saliva mixes with food to allow the food to travel to the stomach easily.

2. As food is being chewed, blood rushes to the digestive system to help the movement of food through it.

3. The gallbladder releases bile into the small intestine, and the pancreas releases digestive enzymes to help with metabolism.

4. Feedback travels back though the vagus nerve, letting you know when you've had enough to eat.

The Three Stages of Digestion

STAGE 1/KAPHA STAGE: Takes place in the mouth, esophagus, and upper part of the stomach

In this stage, predigestive enzymes are at work through our salivary glands that help make the food we are chewing more even and ready to be swallowed. If you're eating too quickly and not chewing food properly, it can result in heartburn, GERD (gastroesophageal reflux disease), and in some cases, ama (leftover food residue) in the digestive tract.

Stage 1 is called the Kapha stage of digestion, due to the saliva production in the mouth (as water is a quality of Kapha).

STAGE 2/PITTA STAGE: Takes place in the lower stomach and small intestine

In this stage, food is broken down to its smallest components by way of acid, bile, and pancreatic secretions. This is where the "heavy lifting" of digestion and metabolism happens, as food is broken down into its smallest components.

Stage 2 is called the Pitta stage of digestion, due to the transformative qualities of gastric juices (bile, stomach acid, digestive enzymes).

STAGE 3/VATA STAGE: Takes place in the large intestine

In this stage, water is removed from the digested food that makes its way to the colon to be eliminated as feces.

Stage 3 is called the Vata stage of digestion, because unusable food matter becomes waste and undergoes a drying process in preparation to be discarded from the body (and drying out is a function of Vata).

It's at this stage that we can start to determine if our bodies are converting food efficiently simply by looking at our stool.

Examining our stool can give us insight into how our digestion is processing food, if the food is of good quality, whether we chewed our food properly, or if there is any ama in our system. It's a way to troubleshoot our metabolic process.

UNDIGESTED FOOD AND THE DISEASE PROCESS

Now we start to see that there some very important factors when it comes to consuming food; choosing to eat foods that are seasonal and/or compatible with our doshas, creating and maintaining healthy digestive and metabolic processes, and chewing our food so it digests correctly to avoid ama production.

Let's take a look at the different types of metabolism related to the three doshas and what can happen when we are out of balance. My favorite analogy when I talk about the digestive fire (agni) is to think if it as a campfire. Building a campfire requires rocks, which represent the digestive system; wood, which represents food to be consumed; and the fire, which represents your agni.

Next, let's look at the type of agni we have and are prone to. Normal agni is the ideal state for all body types and can be achieved by managing stress, eating food in season, and engaging in self-care rituals best for your mind and body type. The wood has been well seasoned and the fire is strong. In the morning, all that remains are the ashes (waste product). No wood is left over (ama), and you can build a new campfire.

HIGH AGNI is when the wood you've used to build your campfire has been soaked in jet-fuel. It burns at a high rate of speed, and you have to add wood constantly to keep the fire burning. The next day, there is nothing left of the wood, and all that remains is burned-out hole in the ground. Even the rocks you used to contain the fire have been scorched. Again, high agni is associated with people who have a predominantly Pitta constitution or imbalance. People with high agni generally don't have much ama in their system, if any, and may be prone to inflammatory digestive disorders (hyperacidity, GERD, and diverticulitis).

VARIABLE AGNI is when the wood used to build your fire is well seasoned and dry, but your fire was built in an area where the wind can strike the flame so that it burns bright or blows out. The next day, most of the wood has been consumed, but there is wood remaining. People with a more Vata constitution or imbalance of Vata will experience moderate ama in the system due to the variability of their agni. Typically, this will result in dry digestive disorders (gas, bloating, and dry stool).

LOW AGNI is when the wood you've used to build your campfire is wet. You need to use a lot of kindling to get the fire started; and once the fire has been lit, the wood has a hard time catching fire. The next day, there is more wood remaining than ash. People who have more of a Kapha constitution or imbalance will experience higher levels of ama in their digestive system because of their sluggish digestion. Typically, this will result in heavy and sluggish digestive disorders (mucous in stool, nausea, and weight gain).

How Do I know if I Have Ama or Not?

There are three symptoms that will present themselves if you do have ama in your system:

1. BAD BREATH: No matter how much you brush, gargle, and chew gum, your breath still smells bad!

2. COATED TONGUE: Typically a sticky white/yellowish coat is present across the surface of your tongue.

3. SHARP BODY ODOR: Typically, more pungent than usual if you naturally have body odor.

The best way to start to dissolve ama in the system is to clean up your diet and lifestyle and to sip hot water throughout the day. You can also reduce the symptoms of ama by oil pulling (gargling and rinsing the mouth with sesame oil), tongue scraping, and dry brushing.

Typically, those who are predominantly Vata and Kapha in nature will be prone to ama, due to their variable and low digestive fire. Ama in Pitta isn't so common, as they will typically have more inflammatory challenges in their digestion.

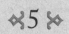

THE
DOSHA
QUIZ

NOW THAT YOU HAVE A BETTER IDEA ABOUT Ayurveda's history, approach, and philosophy, it's time to get a better idea of what your dosha is. You probably already have an idea, and this quiz will give you a better sense of it. I encourage you to be as objective as you can when answering the questions. Keep in mind, though, that this quiz won't tell you the whole story. To be most accurate, get your dosha results by consulting with an Ayurvedic practitioner.

THE GUIDELINES

Circle one or more of the descriptions from each of the categories below—you may fall into one, two, or all three categories.

Add up your results at the bottom of the quiz, and they will give you your dosha.

MY BODY FRAME IS

- A. Slender build, thin boned, some muscle tone
- B. Medium build, athletic, moderate muscle tone
- C. Solid build, large frame, excess muscle or adipose (fat) tissue

MY BODY WEIGHT IS

- A. Low, prominent bones
- B. Moderate, good muscle definition
- C. Heavy, I tend toward weight gain

MY COMPLEXION IS

- A. Dull, dusty, and dry
- B. Rosy, oily, and lustrous
- C. Pale, oily, and smooth

MY SKIN IS

- A. Thin, dry, rough, cold, and cracked
- B. Warm, moist, and freckled
- C. Thick, white, oily, soft, and smooth

MY HAIR IS

- A. Course, dry, brittle, and curly
- B. Moderate, fine, soft, graying or balding
- C. Abundant, oily, and wavy

MY FACE IS

- A. Narrow and oval
- B. Angular and square
- C. Large and round

MY EYES ARE

A. Small, dry, and unsteady

B. Medium, penetrating, and easily irritated

C. Large, watery, and beautiful

MY APPETITE IS

A. Light and variable: I eat like a bird.

B. Voracious and urgent: I can always eat.

C. Consistent and constant: I seem to have constant low-grade hunger.

MY DIGESTION IS

A. Variable; I'm hungry most of the time; sometimes I'm not.

B. Strong; I can digest the kitchen sink!

C. Slow; I sometime feel that my food takes too long to digest.

WHEN IT COMES TO EATING

A. I can skip meals, but can get spacey if I don't eat something eventually. I eat three to five times per day.

B. I cannot skip meals; in fact, I must snack otherwise I get "hangry." I eat five times per day.

C. I can skip meals even though I may feel hungry. I eat two to three times per day.

AFTER EATING MEALS

A. I sometime have gas and am bloated, especially after eating salads or beans.

B. I sometimes experience heartburn or acid reflux, especially after eating spicy foods.

C. I sometimes feel sluggish, especially after eating rich and heavy meals.

WHEN IT COMES TO MY THIRST LEVEL

A. It's moderate; I drink three to six cups of water per day.

B. It's voracious; I need to drink more than eight cups per day.

C. It's low; I tend to retain water and drink three cups per day.

WHEN I POOP

A. It's dry, hard, and I strain. I typically have one bowel movement per day. Sometimes I skip a day.

B. It's medium or loosely formed. They are quick; I'm in and out. I typically have three to four bowel movements per day.

C. They are voluminous. It typically takes me fifteen to twenty minutes to have a bowel movement. I have one bowel movement per day.

MY INTERNAL THERMOSTAT TELLS ME THAT

A. I'm constantly cold. I wear up to four layers—even in the summer. I have cold hands and feet. Brrrrr!

B. I'm always hot. I can sneeze and break a sweat. I run my AC in the winter. Phew!

C. I'm not hot nor cold. I can wear shorts in the fall and early winter. Meh.

WHEN IT COMES TO SOCIAL SITUATIONS, I AM

A. Creative, engaging, and a chatterbox

B. Warm, engaging, and opinionated

C. Quiet, shy, and sometimes aloof

WHEN I LEARN NEW THINGS

A. I'm quick to learn but quick to forget.

B. I'm quick to learn, and will typically know more about something than you do.

C. I'm slow to learn but never forget.

MY SLEEP IS

    A. Irregular and light; I have difficulty getting to sleep and staying asleep.

    B. Light but restful; I typically wake up between 2:00 and 4:00 a.m. to pee but can go back to sleep.

    C. Heavy and deep; I can sleep through an earthquake and love to hit the snooze button on my alarm.

MY EMOTIONAL STATE IS TYPICALLY

    A. Compassionate, anxious, and sometimes fearful

    B. Competitive, irritable, and passionate

    C. Calm, predictable, involved

QUIZ RESULTS

A = Vata total _____

B = Pitta total_____

C = Kapha total_____

My total is_____

That may have been quite eye-opening for you. Perhaps you thought you were a Vata, but you're actually more Kapha. Perhaps you were convinced that you were predominantly Pitta, but your results show that you're an equal mix of Pitta *and* Kapha.

Indeed, it's more likely that when it comes to determining your dosha, you are checking more than one box. Even though most of your answers may fall in the Pitta column, you may have one in Vata and two in Kapha.

It's important to refer to the qualities of each of the doshas and what they do in the body.

WITHOUT VATA, limbs don't move blood and oxygen can't circulate, waste can't be eliminated, and communication (speech as well as at the cellular level) wouldn't occur.

WITHOUT PITTA, you wouldn't be able to metabolize food, your body temperature would fluctuate wildly, and you wouldn't be able process thoughts and experiences.

WITHOUT KAPHA, you would have no structure or form to the body, you wouldn't grow, and you'd have no compassion for others.

Naturally, we tend toward a predominant doaha; however, most people will typically be dual dosha (having a fairly equal combination of two of the doshas).

In traditional Ayurveda, there are seven classical designations of doshic body type.

Mono-dosha (strong predominance of one dosha)

>   Vata   Pitta   Kapha

Dual-dosha (predominance of one dosha with an almost equal mix of another) This is what most people are.

>   Pitta/Vata   Pitta/Kapha   Kapha/Vata

Tri-dosha (equal mix of all three doshas)

>   Vata   Pitta   Kapha

Tri-doshas are quite rate. Possibly only 5 percent of the global population is Tri-doshic, and the people are either balanced all the time with little fluctuation or a complete hot mess and constantly trying to come back into balance.

What's important to remember about your body type (also called *Prakruti*, or the constitution you're born with) is that it doesn't change over your lifetime. Prakruti is the inherent ideal balance of the doshas. Health is the state of Prakruti.

If you were born a Pitta/Kapha, you will be a Pitta/Kapha for the rest of your life. The only thing that will change is your state of balance (also called Vikruti). Vikruti is the nature of imbalance. Virkruti describes the doshas in their current state—disease is the state of Vikruti.

The keyword to balancing your dosha lies in the qualities of your dosha. For example, if you're Pitta/Vata, you want to balance the heat, mobility, and oily qualities of Pitta, as well as the dry, light, and mobile qualities of Vata. Too much air from Vata can cause the fire in Pitta to burn hotter or burn out! Remember, like increases like, and it's important to understand how your doshas go out of balance and how to bring them back to balance before the imbalance gets worse.

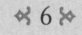

AYURVEDIC
NUTRITION

IN WESTERN NUTRITION, WE LOOK AT THE ELEMENTS of food based on their nutritional qualities: carbohydrates (simple and complex), fats, proteins, and sugars. We know that consuming more protein will help us build more muscle, that eating more sugar or simple carbohydrates will give us more energy if we are active or make us gain weight if we are not, and that we typically have a love/hate relationship with foods that are high in fat.

Another practice of Western nutrition is the broad categorization of foods based on a general understanding of what we "should" be consuming and how much. This can be found in the now-retired food pyramid that we are all taught in grade school.

Personally, I never understood this concept for two reasons: 1) I always felt sick if I ate too many complex carbs (the foods at the base of the food pyramid), and 2) that pyramids were for pharaohs, not food. Of course, we are now aware that many people have food intolerances and allergies to things like gluten, dairy, and soy, so the food pyramid no longer works for all of us equally.

The Ayurvedic approach to nutrition is different, because we look at the qualities of foods as well as the nutritional benefits based on their elemental qualities, which are similar to the elemental qualities of the three doshas.

Food is data—it has a physical and an emotional reaction on our physiology. By understanding the elemental qualities of the foods we consume, we can start to understand what effects we will experience after consuming them.

Each of the six tastes can increase, be neutral to, or decrease the doshas. In Ayurveda, food is used as medicine, so understanding how the food you're eating affects your body is key to balancing your health.

THE SIX TASTES (RASA)

The six tastes of Ayurveda are sweet, sour, salty, pungent, bitter, and astringent. In addition to having an effect on our mind and body chemistry, our body uses food to build, repair, and replace tissues. As each of the six tastes is governed by the five elements, the quantity and quality of certain foods will also have an effect on the development and replenishment of the tissues based on their elemental qualities.

SWEET: The taste of sweet contains the elements of earth and water. The body uses foods that are classified as sweet in nature to build and bulk tissues and help calm nerves. Therefore, sweet foods can increase imbalances of Kapha (water and earth), and reduce Vata and

Pitta, as sweet foods are inherently cold, damp, and heavy by nature.

EXAMPLES OF SWEET FOODS: milk, dried fruit, beets, rice, and bread

SOUR: The taste of sour contains the elements of earth and fire. The body uses foods that are classified as sour in nature to cleanse tissues and increase mineral absorption. Therefore, sour foods can increase imbalances of Pitta (fire and water) and Kapha (water) and reduce Vata, as sour foods are hot, damp, and heavy by nature.

EXAMPLES OF SOUR FOODS: yogurt, pickles, lemons, wine, and fermented foods

SALTY: The taste of salty contains the elements of earth and water. The body uses foods that are classified as salty in nature to improve the taste of food, lubricate the tissues, and stimulate digestion. Therefore, salty foods can increase imbalances of Pitta (fire) and Kapha (earth) and reduce Vata, as salty foods are hot, damp, and heavy by nature. However, salty foods in excess can dry out Vata.

EXAMPLES OF SALTY FOODS: sea salt, sea vegetables, and celery

PUNGENT: The taste of pungent contains the elements of fire and air. The body uses foods that are classified as pungent in nature to stimulate digestion and increase metabolism. Therefore, pungent foods can increase imbalances of Pitta (fire) and Vata (air), and reduce Kapha, as pungent foods are hot, dry, and light by nature.

EXAMPLES OF PUNGENT FOODS: garlic, onions, ginger, and chile peppers

BITTER: The taste of bitter contains the elements of air and space. The body uses foods that are classified as bitter in nature to detoxify and lighten tissues. Therefore, bitter foods can increase imbalances of Vata (air and space) and reduce Pitta and Kapha, as bitter foods are cold, dry, and light by nature.

EXAMPLES OF BITTER FOODS: turmeric, kale, spinach, and olives

ASTRINGENT: The taste of astringent contains the elements of air and space. The body uses foods that are classified as astringent in nature to absorb water, tone tissues, and reduce inflammation. Therefore, astringent foods can increase imbalances of Vata (air and space) and reduce Pitta and Kapha, as bitter foods are cold, dry, and light by nature.

EXAMPLES OF ASTRINGENT FOODS: legumes, pears, pomegranates, and apples

Sweet foods increase Kapha and reduce Vata and Pitta.
Sour foods increase Kapha and Pitta and reduce Vata.
Salty foods increase Kapha and Pitta and reduce Vata.
Pungent foods increase Vata and Pitta and reduce Kapha.
Bitter foods increase Vata and reduce Pitta and Kapha.
Astringent foods increase Vata and reduce Pitta and Kapha.

FOOD MINDFULNESS (SADHANA)

In addition to understanding how to eat the six tastes in order to have a strong digestion, we also have to be mindful about how we cook, handle, and consume foods.

Imbalances can be brought on by eating too quickly, eating while working on other projects, being distracted, being angry or upset when cooking, or eating food that is too old or has too many preservatives.

Every time I work with a new patient, part of the unique program I create for the patient includes the food mindfulness list. In some cases, just engaging with food in a more mindful way greatly helps a person's digestion and metabolism become stronger.

FOOD MINDFULNESS LIST

1. Eat in the proper place (sitting at a table).
2. Eat food prepared by loving hands in a loving way.
3. Give gratitude before meals.
4. Eat without distraction (don't drive, work, or watch TV while eating).
5. Eat in a relaxed frame of mind—if you're stressed or anxious, don't eat.
6. Chew food until it is at an even consistency; don't inhale your food.
7. Prefer warm food to cold when possible.
8. Avoid leftovers (food that is more than three days old may cause illness).
9. Choose food that is oily or moist, because dry food is harder to digest.
10. Drink only a small amount of liquid with meals, because too much liquid can dilute gastric juices.
11. Avoid ice-cold drinks; ice water causes the digestion to come to a grinding halt.
12. Eat with self-confidence, even if it's a chocolate bar.
13. Eat until you are only two-thirds full—overeating may leave undigested food in the system.
14. Rest after eating, 5–8 minutes minimum.
15. Allow three hours between meals; this allows the digestive process to happen.

Even if you're able to incorporate only some of these into your routine, you may find a profound change in how your body digests your food. Finding gratitude is one of the subtle teachings in Ayurveda and in yoga, and it can positively impact your health.

7

HOW WE GET SICK: A CLOSER LOOK AT STRESS IN THE DISEASE PROCESS

THE ABILITY TO MANAGE AND REDUCE OUR stress levels directly impacts every system in our body, starting with our digestive system. The longer we are stressed and don't have a way to reduce or remove stress from our system, the deeper an imbalance can go, making it harder to come back to balance.

We are subject to two types of stress:

"GOOD" STRESS: EUSTRESS

Eustress provides motivation for us to live a more productive life and gives us a sense of purpose and responsibility in life.

- ❁ Helps us adapt to change and evolution
- ❁ Helps us perform tasks better and more efficiently
- ❁ Protects us by "fight, flight, or freeze"
- ❁ Improves creativity and productivity

"BAD" STRESS: DISTRESS

Distress is stress that is a result of trauma or that has accumulated over time, hasn't been reduced or removed, and keeps us in fight, flight, or freeze.

❁ Emotional/situational stress from work, family, and relationships

❁ Long periods of stress without stress-reducing techniques

❁ Stress due to physical or emotional illness

HOW TO BETTER MANAGE YOUR STRESS

In my experience, one of the leading factors in imbalances and disease comes from an accumulation of stress and the inability to reduce or remove stress from our system.

Consider how you currently manage your stress. Do you have a yoga practice or meditation ritual? Do you maintain an exercise program like running or swimming? Perhaps you like to take a hot bath in times of stress. These are all very good stress-reducing techniques; however, when you need an immediate reduction in stress, chances are, you're looking for stress-reducing experience that will release dopamine in the brain through one or more of the five senses.

Out of the five senses, the sense of taste is one of the most powerful senses we have. When we encounter stress, we often look to food for emotional support to get us through challenging situations related to work, family, and relationships as well as life-changing events like the sudden loss of a friend or loved one.

Stress eating is something we all have experienced in our lives, and the more we engage in stress eating as a tool to manage our stress, the harder our bodies have to work to come back into balance.

TIME AND THE JUSTIFICATION OF "BAD" BEHAVIORS

How long we go without acknowledging that something may be wrong with us impacts our health. When we ignore the symptoms of an impending imbalance and "power through," we can actually get considerably sicker. The longer we force ourselves to power through situations and not focus on the root of the problem, the harder it is to treat and cure our imbalance.

Let's look at how we get sick. First are the coping mechanisms we engage in when encountering a stressful situation, as well as the frequency of those situations in our lives. Let's say you eat a balanced diet, manage your stress well by going to yoga classes three times a week, get out into nature every weekend, and don't bring your work home with you. Suddenly, your boss asks you to take on a very exciting project that is not only something you've wanted to work on but that will surely put you in line for a promotion. Your hours start to get longer, your yoga practice goes to twice a week (when you can make it), you spend the weekends at the office, and some of your meals come from the vending machine. This is step one to getting sick.

As the project ramps up even more, you're tasked with more responsibility and fewer resources, late hours, and all-weekend work. Your yoga practice dwindles to "once in a blue moon," your meals are regularly foraged from the vending machine, your coffee consumption is up to five cups per day, and the quality and duration of your sleep begin to suffer. This is step two to getting sick.

As the project comes to it end, you start feeling drained. Your bowels are erratic, you've been fighting a cold for four weeks in a row, you're not sleeping, you may be consuming alcohol to help you sleep, your typical meal consists of candy and potato chips, and you're more emotional toward people. This is step three to getting sick, and you now have a choice—you can "power through" or ask for a break. That can be a massage, a much-needed day off, or possibly the option to delegate some parts of your project to other people. If you don't do anything at all, you'll be entering step four of getting sick.

Step four is when the body, which happens to be way smarter then you, *forces* you to take time off because now you have a full-blown illness that makes it impossible for you to do anything but stay at home. This can be as mild as a head cold or the flu or can become something more serious and long lasting. It all depends on your body's ability to bounce back, family genetics, and whether you've had a previous infection, illness, or injury.

BIOLOGICAL AND LINEAR TIME THE IN DISEASE PROCESS

Let's look at the actual time it takes us to get sick: biological time versus linear time. The longer and more frequently you engage in poor habits and lifestyle choices to cope with stress, the faster and more often you'll experience an imbalance.

Vata

Because of their "lighter" body type, people who are predominantly Vata will experience a shorter duration of distress before their body goes out of balance.

Some typical conditions that can cause an imbalance of Vata are

- Cold, dry, and blustery weather
- Consuming dry and cold foods, like salads and chips
- Poor sleep hygiene and not being able to rest
- Excessive air travel
- Excessive worry and anxiety

You can experience a Vata imbalance even if your primary dosha is Pitta or Kapha.

If you are predominantly Vata, however, you may experience these imbalances more frequently and in a more moderate to severe way:

- Dry skin
- Poor circulation
- Gas and bloating
- Scattered thoughts

Pitta

As Pittas are intense and driven, people who are predominantly Pitta in nature will experience a moderate duration of distress before experiencing an imbalance.

Some typical conditions that can cause an imbalance of Pitta are

- ❀ Hot and muggy weather conditions

- ❀ Excess consumption of spicy and oily foods, alcohol, and red meat

- ❀ Excess exposure to the sun

- ❀ Overthinking/"monkey mind"

- ❀ Being in constant competition with self and others

Pitta imbalance can also occur in people with a primary dosha of Vata or Kapha.

If you are predominantly Pitta, however, you may experience these imbalances more frequently and in a more moderate-to-severe way:

- ❀ Hyperacidity
- ❀ Skin rashes

- ❀ Excessive heat/hot flashes
- ❀ Anger issues

Kapha

Kaphas are more solid and slower-moving than Vatas and Pittas, and because of their slower and stoic nature will experience a longer duration in distress before experiencing an imbalance.

Typical conditions that can cause an imbalance of Kapha are

- ❀ Cold and damp weather conditions

- ❀ Excess consumption of rich, heavy, and oily foods

- ❀ Lack of exercise/preference for hibernation

- ❀ Being overly attached to people and possessions

- ❀ Withdrawing from friends and social situations

A Kapha imbalance can also occur in people with a primary dosha of Vata or Pitta.

If you are predominantly Kapha, however, you may experience these imbalances more frequently and in a more moderate-to-severe way:

- ❀ **Weight gain**
- ❀ **Acne**
- ❀ **Lethargy**
- ❀ **Depression**

MANAGING STRESS WITH FOOD

When we eat to cope with a distressing situation, we are relying on food to soothe us by releasing a shot of dopamine (the feel-good hormone) in our brain. This signals that we are "rewarding" ourselves and managing our stressful situation; however, the food choices we make to get that "reward" may not be the best choice to keep our health balanced.

Eating when we are encountering distress can also lead to several digestive and physiological challenges, including weight gain, ama production, lethargy, and illness. When we are in a state of distress, our psoas muscles (also known as our fight or flight muscles because they activate when we are stressed) are firing, our adrenals are online, and our breathing becomes shallow as we prepare to fight or run. It takes a considerable amount of blood to prepare our body to fight or flee. It also takes a considerable amount of blood to move food through the digestive system. There isn't enough blood to do both.

When we reduce our stress, even just by simply taking ten deep breaths, our metabolic process increases. This reduces the threat of poor digestion, malabsorption, and ama production in the digestive tract as well as our risk of an imbalance.

SPOTTING IMBALANCE EARLY AND REGAINING BALANCE

The signs of an imbalance are subtle, but one way we can determine if we are stressed is what types of foods we are craving. As taste is one of the most powerful of our five senses, it's typically our first line of defense against stress. The rituals surrounding food are part of our patterned behavior, as well as how we "justify" our food choices and consumption. Remember, food is data, and how you eat based on how you feel will always let you know if you're eating foods that can cause harm or encourage healing. In Ayurveda, like increases like!

Vata

First sign of an imbalance: Gas, bloating, and dry stool

Second sign of an imbalance: Scattered thoughts and anxiety

Vatagenic foods: Foods that are dry, light, and cold in nature will cause an increase of Vata. Salads and raw vegetables, crackers, chips, iced foods (smoothies), granola, kale chips, dried nuts, and diets low in fats

Additionally, eating foods "on-the-go" and irregularly will also increase Vata.

Pitta

First sign of an imbalance: Loose bowels, diarrhea, and reflux

Second sign of an imbalance: Judgmental behavior and anger

Pittagenic foods: Foods that are hot, oily, and sharp (sour) in nature will cause an increase of Pitta. Additionally, eating foods too quickly or when stressed will also increase Pitta.

Tomatoes, peppers, eggplant, red meat, spicy foods, cabbage, kombucha, alcohol, greasy foods, excessive oil, and nut butters

Kapha

First sign of an imbalance: Sluggish digestion, mucus in stool, and lethargy

Second sign of an imbalance: Obsessive thoughts, withdrawal from social connections

Kaphagenic foods: Foods that are cold, heavy, and oily in nature will cause an increase of Kapha. Additionally, eating too frequently and consuming heavy and rich meals will also increase Kapha.

Dairy (cheese, milk, ice cream), pastas, breads, deep-fried foods, candy, excessively oily food, and processed/convenience foods

THE COMPUTER ANALOGY

The human body experiences life through the five senses. Essentially these are data ports to the body; and our body digests, metabolizes, and "processes" the data from these inputs. These five data ports allow us to interact with others and experience the world around us but can cause us to go out of balance if experienced in excess. We process what we see and how to discern what we are seeing with our eyes. We process what we are hearing and listen to sound with our ears. We process heat and cold, rough and smooth with our skin. We process taste and flavor with our tongue and mouth, and we process smell and aroma with our nose.

Now, take a look at your computer; it too has five data inputs: the power port, WiFi, Bluetooth, a USB port, and an SD card. The computer interacts with the data on these inputs and processes it as needed—the same way we interact and process data through our five senses. If the data is good and the computer is functioning optimally it typically won't slow down, freeze, or falter. However, if the data coming into the computer is of poor quality—for example, if it has a worm or virus or is incompatible with the computer—the data will cause the computer to run slowly, causing a lag in completing other tasks. Over time, not cleaning the hard drive or running an anti-virus program will cause the computer to be unable to process data anymore and will require major repairs.

It's the same with the human body—the more we encounter incompatible "data," the harder our body has to work to "process" it.

As food has the biggest influence on our physiology and is a necessity for us to live, much of our "incompatible data" comes from the foods we consume. Naturally, this will be different for everyone: some of us crave sweet foods, some of us crave salty, some crave oily, and some crave dry.

Eating foods that take us out of balance isn't too bad for us if we consume them on a moderate basis, but if we eat these types of foods on a more regular basis, they can cause our "hard drive" (digestive system) to max out and slow down.

It's important to know that our digestive system influences all other systems in our body because it produces the tissues that interact with those systems. Remember, we are what we metabolize, and much like poor quality food causes the digestive system to become upset, if the tissues produced from the metabolic process are of poor quality, they will cause that specific system to go out of balance, causing more long-term health challenges.

SIX STAGES OF DISEASE

Even though Vata is the only "mobile" dosha, each of the doshas is constantly reacting to all of your inputs (stress, food, alcohol, and other things that cause imbalance). Remember, the definition of dosha is "that which can cause harm or become faulty," so keep your doshas balanced to avoid imbalance, which can manifest in sickness or disease.

From the Ayurvedic perspective, disease has a total of six stages of development:

1. Accumulation
2. Aggravation
3. Overflow
4. Relocation
5. Manifestation
6. Diversification

And circling back to my teacher saying, "water the root to enjoy the fruit," let's use my tree analogy to describe the disease process better.

ACCUMULATION and **AGGRAVATION** occur in the digestive system and can be prevented from going deeper into the body by understanding our self-referral. In the tree analogy, these two stages occur in the roots of the tree. By tending to the essential needs of the tree (water quality, sunlight, plant food, and so on) these two phases can retreat, and the tree stays healthy. These first two stages function as our "early warning" system. As we learn to identify our imbalances at these early stages of disease development through self-referral, we can help alleviate them, and our system will return to homeostasis.

If the doshas are not balanced in the accumulation or aggravation phases, they will overflow into the body, either by hitching a ride in the blood or plasma (the "waters" of the body), continuing the disease process into the third stage of disease, known as **OVERFLOW**. In the tree analogy, disease overflows from the roots and finds a ride in the sap of the tree.

At this point, the doshas become predatory and will circulate through the body until they locate a weak area in the tissues or in an organ where they will take up residence. This is the fourth step in disease pathology, called **RELOCATION**. In the tree analogy, disease has found a weakened branch and begins to move in.

The fifth step in disease development is called **MANIFESTATION**. In this phase, the dosha becomes more comfortable in its new home, and the symptoms that are associated with the energetic disturbance

of the tissues or organ will deepen. During this phase, the characteristics of the disease are codified, and allopathic medicine gives the
disease or infection a name. Pharmaceutical or surgical treatments
may be administered. In the tree analogy, the disease begins pre-
senting as abnormalities in the bark and leaves. Treatments may be
administered and the tree may be pruned or cut back to prevent the
disease from spreading.

The sixth and final step in the disease process is called DIVER-
SIFICATION. During this final stage, symptoms become quite specific to the affected site and are very pronounced and severe. Tissues
and organs that have been infiltrated by the imbalanced dosha may
become irreparably damaged. If diversification occurs in a vital organ,
a transplant may need to be considered or more invasive surgery may
be needed. Pharmaceutical protocols are either not useful or are just
managing the severe symptoms of disease. In extreme cases, the host
may succumb to the disease. In the tree analogy, the disease has infiltrated every part of the tree; blossoms and fruit (if fruit-bearing) are
compromised, and the tree will be cut down to prevent the disease
from spreading to other trees.

Preventing disease starts in our digestive system—also known
in Ayurveda as the "inner disease pathway." It's in this system
that our tissues are formed, so if we experience an imbalance and
don't address it in the first two stages of disease development, the
imbalance can affect how our tissues are formed.

8

YOU ARE WHAT YOU EAT: FOOD, METABOLISM, AND TISSUE DEVELOPMENT

DIGESTION AND METABOLISM FROM THE Ayurvedic perspective can be a bit complex, but they are easily broken down into steps:

You now know that digestion starts in the mouth and upper part of the stomach. This is called stage 1 or the Kapha stage.

Stage 2, or the Pitta stage of digestion, takes place in the lower part of the stomach and the small intestine. This is where the heavy lifting of digestion takes place and our "primary" agni comes into play. This agni, responsible for digestion, is called JATHARAGNI.

Jatharagni has two functions; the first is to convert food into predigested absorbable nutrients in preparation for further metabolizing. It also kills certain types of foodborne pathogens. The second function of Jatharagni is regulating the temperature of the body.

If we are consuming foods that are hard to digest or if we aren't chewing properly, the Jatharagni has to work much harder to break food down before it can go into micro-digestion. In this case, Vatas may experience lethargy and drowsiness. Pittas may experience acid reflux and, in some cases, sweating. Kaphas may experience sluggishness.

The digestive process continues in the small intestine with the help of the liver and pancreas, and that's where the metabolic magic truly happens. Yes, our body is breaking down food to give us energy, but, according to the system of Ayurveda, it's also where our tissues are made, and how, over the course of thirty to thirty-five days, our body will replenish, refresh, and replace the worn-out tissues with new ones.

THE SEVEN TISSUES (DHATUS) OF THE BODY AND HOW THEY ARE FORMED

Each tissue is made during Stage 2 of digestion, or the Pitta stage. Each tissue is governed by one of the five elements:

- ❀ **Lymph (Rasa): Governed by water; found in the lymphatic system**
- ❀ **Blood (Rakta): Governed by fire; found in the circulatory system**
- ❀ **Muscle (Mamsa): Governed by earth; found in the muscular system**
- ❀ **Fat (Medas): Governed by water; found in the integumentary system**
- ❀ **Bones (Ashti): Governed by earth; found in the skeletal system**
- ❀ **Nerves (Majja): Governed by air; found in the nervous system**
- ❀ **Ovum/Sperm (Shukra): Governed by water; found in in the reproductive and endocrine systems**

Imagine that your entire digestive system is an industrial manufacturing park with seven factories in a row. Each of these factories produces one of the seven bodily tissues from the food you have consumed. Imagine the food you've consumed has to pass through each of the factories that are producing each of the seven tissues.

As your tissues are made in succession, the first stop is at the factory that produces lymph (Rasa). Here, the lymph tissue is made from the food. Once the lymph manufacturing process is complete and the unusable material has been discarded, the food goes on to the next step in the manufacturing process, which is to the factory that produces blood (Rakta). Once the blood tissue has been made and the unusable material has been discarded, the food goes onto the next step in the manufacturing process, which is where the muscle tissue (Mamsa) is made. The same process happens in the factories that produce fat, bone, nerve, and reproductive tissue, until the food has been used up, and all the waste has been transported to the large intestine and bladder for waste removal.

In order for high-quality tissues to be made, the manufacturing process is dependent on high-quality raw material (food) and the efficiency of the previous factory. For example, if the factory producing lymph tissue is not functioning optimally and produces poor quality lymph due to an imbalance in the digestive system, all subsequent tissues will be compromised, until the imbalance can be fixed.

So, if the digestive system is essentially a factory for producing tissues through the metabolic (or manufacturing) process, we know that there are certain conditions needed in order for our tissues to be made of the highest quality:

1. Strong agni
2. Little or no ama
3. Consumption of high-quality/compatible food
4. Not eating while distracted; not eating at odd hours
5. Doshas in balance

WHAT HAPPENS TO OUR TISSUES WHEN THERE IS AN IMBALANCE OF A DOSHA?

When it comes to the quality and quantity of our tissues, the state of balance with our doshas is very important. We already know that Vata is light, dry, and mobile by nature. We know that Pitta is hot, sharp, and intense by nature; and we know that Kapha is oily, heavy, and soft by nature. Any increase of Vata, Pitta, or Kapha in our manufacturing process will cause these qualities of our tissues to suffer the impact of our imbalance.

Excess Vata

When there is too much Vata in the tissue manufacturing process, the tissues produced will be minimal in quantity. The form and function of the tissue will be weak and prone to injury and harder to repair if damage is repetitive.

Excess Pitta

When there is too much Pitta in the tissue manufacturing process, the tissues produced will be moderate in quantity. The tissues will be strong in quality but will be prone to inflammation.

Excess Kapha

When there is too much Kapha in the tissue manufacturing process, the tissues produced will be excessive in quantity and hard and inflexible in quality.

If a dosha has infiltrated one or more of the tissues, bringing the body back into balance will be more complex and will take longer than if we catch it before it goes farther.

Other factors like our age, the time of year, and how long we've been out of balance can make the path to balance harder and longer, which is why many of us "give up" on preventative treatments and seek modern medicine to manage symptoms. Just remember, it took a long time for you to go out of balance, so it's going to take some time for you to return to balance. As I tell my yoga students: the journey to balance is the destination.

We already know that that having weak or variable agni may cause the production of ama, which will impact how our tissues are created. We have also established that the consumption of poor-quality or incompatible foods will also impact how our tissues are formed.

ANABOLIC METABOLISM VERSUS CATABOLIC METABOLISM

When we consume foods, our body goes through two different types of metabolism: the first is catabolism, or catabolic metabolism. Catabolic metabolism is also known as the "destructive" metabolism. What happens in catabolic metabolism is our body takes the nutrients from food (plants and animals) and breaks down these substances into simpler ones, with the release of energy. Catabolic metabolism is also known as macro-digestion.

The second is anabolism, or anabolic metabolism. Anabolic metabolism is the constructive metabolism, in which our body takes the nutrients from our food and synthesizes more complex substances from simpler ones, which can be used to replenish the tissues of our body. This is also known as micro-digestion.

When we are eating while distracted (emailing, driving, watching TV, reading) we aren't able to be present with the food we're eating and, therefore, may not chew it properly. Another issue is eating meals at irregular times. We sometimes tend to barely have breakfast, eat lunch over our keyboards between noon and 2:00 p.m., and consume a large meal between 7:00 and 9:00 p.m. before heading to bed between 11:00 p.m. and midnight, which typically makes digestion very hard, as the body is preparing for rest, and we are asking that the "factory" wake up and start producing tissues. Typically, if you're waking up between 2:00 and 4:00 a.m. with night sweats and heartburn, you probably ate too late.

DOSHIC TIME AND CIRCADIAN RHYTHMS

Each of the doshas governs certain times of the day and night. Being in harmony with these times is not always possible, as we may work long hours, skip meals, and have too many late night activities we enjoy. However, a good day starts with a good night's sleep.

During the morning phase of Kapha, rise by 6:00 a.m. and engage in your morning rituals, especially if you're more Kapha in nature.

- ❊ Empty your bowels and bladder
- ❊ Practice yoga asana
- ❊ Drink hot water and ginger
- ❊ Enjoy breakfast

During the evening Kapha phase, we prepare for rest. Eat a light meal by 7:00 p.m., and be in bed with the lights out by 10:00 p.m.

PITTA TIME: 10:00 A.M.–2:00 P.M./10:00 P.M.–2:00 A.M.

During the morning/afternoon phase of Pitta, we are typically at work. It's the most productive time. Stop at noon to have lunch.

- ❊ If you feel hungry, eat
- ❊ Consume your largest meal between noon–1:00 p.m.
- ❊ Take a few minutes to rest or walk after your meal

During the night/early morning Pitta phase, you are resting and digesting your food. Eating late can give heartburn or acid reflux between midnight and 2:00 a.m., especially to more Pitta natures.

VATA TIME: 2:00 A.M.–6:00 A.M./2:00 P.M.–6:00 P.M.

During the afternoon/evening phase of Vata time, you may feel tired, especially if you haven't taken a break or if you've eaten lunch at your desk. You may feel hungry if lunch was light or not sustaining.

- ❊ Enjoy a snack with tea
- ❊ If you feel tired, stand up and stretch or take a 5–10 minute walk
- ❊ Avoid cookies or high-caffeine drinks; they will impact your sleep

During the early morning Vata phase, your body is in an active dream state and preparing waste products for elimination. You may need to urinate between 2:00 a.m. and 4:00 a.m.

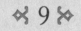

BALANCING
YOUR DOSHA

BALANCE DOESN'T HAPPEN OVERNIGHT. THERE IS no magic pill—only your patience and perseverance in evolving your habits and tendencies. With these suggestions, it's important that you start with two to three recommendations at a time, rather than attempting to do them all at once. You may find that you'll never leave your house if you do! It can take up to three weeks to incorporate new practices and rituals into your routine before they become habits, so start where you are and move at your own pace!

I always suggest bringing your primary care practitioner into the conversation as you start any new lifestyle protocol. As you come back into balance, your health care provider may need to adjust any medications you might be taking, and it's always a good idea to keep your team in the loop.

HOW TO BALANCE VATA

Vata imbalances occur when there is excess dryness, lightness, movement, cold, and variability.

The first sign of a Vata imbalance typically starts in the digestive system and may present as excessive gas and distension (especially after eating) and stools that are drier and harder than normal and less frequent. Excess Vata can also cause a feeling of being less grounded, as well as more anxious.

FACTORS CONTRIBUTING TO A VATA IMBALANCE ARE

- Excessive travel
- Excessive work schedule/too much on your plate
- Excessive consumption of dry and light foods (salads, nuts, dried fruit, granola, chips, and crackers)
- Excessive consumption of cold foods (smoothies, iced foods and drinks)
- Lack of good-quality oils in the diet
- Highly variable routine
- Poor sleep hygiene (due to excessive worry)
- Cold and/or dry climate
- Vata season (late fall to mid-to-late winter)

Vata governs communication, transportation, and elimination in the body. It allows you to communicate with others as air passes through your vocal cords. It is the force that allows nerve impulses to occur. It allows your blood to cycle through your body and air to pass into and out of your lungs; it governs the waste removal process in your body; and it helps with your creative and artistic tendencies.

Of all three doshas, Vata is the only one that is mobile—Pitta and Kapha are unmoving. This is because of Vata's combination of space and air. It also means that Vata, truly the only dynamic dosha, causes fire to burn, water to flow, and earth to solidify and is typically the culprit behind imbalances in the body. Vata does not just cause imbalances of Vata, but of Pitta and Kapha as well.

Vatas are creative, ethereal, and erudite. They are the friend you have with a deeply creative mind, as well as the one who possesses much knowledge about a wide variety of topics, from art and science to geography and history. Vatas are truly inspiring, imaginative, and playful when in balance but can be anxious, scattered, unstable, and erratic when out of balance.

Conversations that are typically creative and informed can become sporadic and incoherent when a Vata is imbalanced. If they've taken on too many projects or if they are feeling overwhelmed in a relationship or professional situation, Vatas tend to become like a butterfly in a hurricane.

You know you're a Vata when you realize that you are the one with a permanently full voicemail, have thirty-five unanswered texts, and only use your email "sparingly" because it can be overwhelming to receive all of those newsletters you signed up for. If you're a Vata, the best way to contact you may be through your social media platforms, where you are completely up-to-date with everything and everyone. You think about how to respond to certain communications. In fact, it may take you five or six versions of a text or email before you're happy with it, and that's only after you've slept on it for a few days. You read and post tweets and Instagram posts thoroughly and frequently, however.

Diet and lifestyle recommendations for Vata aren't about preventing the wind from blowing; they are more about mastering the hurricane of variability and preventing the Vata from being swept up in the tornado called life. When it comes to balancing yourself through diet and lifestyle edits, remember, rituals *are* good things, and you can still be a free spirit even if you practice a small routine to keep yourself balanced. Routines can be of great benefit to your mind and body balance. Start with one of the recommendations—maybe two—and stick to them. They won't cramp your style, I promise.

VATA EVENING RITUALS FOR BETTER SLEEP

1. Stop using all blue-screen devices (cell phone, tablet, computer, and television) at least forty-five minutes before bedtime.

2. Set your thermostat in cold weather to be 70°F about ten minutes before your wake-up time. This will ensure your house is warm when you rise.

3. Use a humidifier in the colder and dryer months.

4. Brush and floss your teeth and scrape your tongue.

5. Get into bed by 10:00 p.m., and in the winter, use a hot water bottle to warm the bed before you get into it.

6. Massage your feet with organic sesame oil or a high-quality foot cream, paying special attention to the soles of your feet. Spend at least five minutes on each foot. Wear cotton socks on your feet after the massage—especially if you are using sesame oil.

7. Take ten deep belly breaths to reduce your heart rate and settle your mind and body.

8. Use silicone ear plugs if your partner snores or if you live in a busy city.

9. Turn your lights out by 10:15 p.m.

1. Rise and shine by 6:00 a.m. Don't linger in bed checking emails or social media.

2. Drink hot water with freshly grated ginger or ginger tea. If you consume coffee, have the ginger tea first.

3. Meditate for 10–20 minutes. This can be a meditation of choice—of which there are so many. There are several good ones in *A Little Bit of Meditation* by Amy Leigh Mercree.

4. Practice some pranayama (breathing exercise).

5. Practice a yoga asana for 20–30 minutes.

6. Dry-brush before showering. Dry brushing not only helps remove dead skin cells but also helps bring circulation back to the skin. To dry-brush, start with a soft, natural bristle brush. Making circular motions, start with your feet and work your way up your legs, stomach, arms, and back—avoid the heart. This process can take 8–10 minutes.

7. Oil pulling. As part of your oral health ritual, use 1–2 tablespoons of organic sesame and swish the oil around your mouth for 15 to 20 minutes. Oil pulling can help reduce ama in your digestive system, reduce dryness in the mouth, and help improve digestion. If you're feeling extra industrious, you can oil pull as you're dry brushing! Do not swallow the oil! Spit the oil/saliva mix into paper cup or a trash bag and cover it with a napkin or paper towel to absorb the oil.

8. Take a warm shower or bath. Make sure the water isn't too hot, as it can dry out your skin. When dry, apply moisturizer all over your body, including hands, face, and feet.

9. Use a nourishing soap or body wash.

10. In cold weather, make sure you wear enough layers to stay warm throughout the day.

11. Eat a hot breakfast with high-quality oils. For example, this could be oatmeal with ghee, honey, and cinnamon; basmati rice and an egg with ghee and black pepper; or avocado on toast. If you are craving a smoothie, avoid anything iced, and remember to chew it (you can just swish the liquid around your mouth like mouthwash).

12. Make sure you have healthy emergency snacks with you—cashews, almonds, and nutrition bars that aren't dry are good options. But remember, these are for emergency use ONLY!

13. Plan your meals. Consume your largest meal at lunch, and avoid distractions while you eat (no email or TV, no driving, and so on).

Moderate your salad consumption—especially in the late fall and winter months.

14. **Find your routine.** Even though Vatas like to fly by the seat of their pants, there is something to be said for having a little structure in your life. One good place to start is with a weekly activity that you can do with friends (yoga class, hiking, knitting).

15. **Favor warm and cooked foods whenever possible**, and make sure the foods you're eating are made with high-quality oils, like ghee, olive oil, or sesame oil.

16. **Be active, be busy, AND know your limitations and when to say no.** Even though you may LOVE being involved with many different projects, when you get overwhelmed, you tend to procrastinate; and in the end, your work may be rushed, messy, or mediocre.

17. **Keep a gratitude journal of all that you are grateful for.** This can be your family and friends or even that nice person who bought you a cup of coffee randomly today. Be grateful. Having gratitude is a great way to keep your heart open.

Food and Eating Plan for Vata

Most people who are predominantly Vata typically eat light meals (when they remember to eat). On a "good day," Vatas may eat a large salad for lunch or dinner. On a more challenging day, Vatas will eat whatever convenience foods are in arm's reach (cookies, crackers, and other snacks). As we've discussed, excessive consumption of Vatagenic foods (salads, cookies, crackers) will cause Vata to go out of balance. It's important for Vatas to consume meals that are well cooked with high-quality oils, especially in the winter and early spring months (Vata season). That means that it's advisable not only to follow a food schedule but also to incorporate some meal planning into your routine. This may be challenging, as most Vatas prefer to "go with the flow" rather than plan; however, planning is part of the therapy to balance Vata.

Vata Food Schedule

7:00-7:30 A.M. Enjoy a cooked breakfast. Your digestion has to wake up and turn on, so it's important to give it food that is easily digested. If you are a green smoothie fan, consume it as a snack at 10:00 a.m.; just hold the ice (and that includes frozen fruit).

10:00-10:30 A.M. If you start to feel a little grumble in your stomach, have a snack. This can be some fruit, almonds (raw, not roasted or salted), or a small muffin. You can also have some tea at this point as well. If you aren't hungry, don't eat.

NOON-1:00 P.M. This is when you have your biggest meal of the day, and don't make it a huge salad. You need sustenance, and eating a salad everyday can cause Vata to increase and eventually go out of balance. Let's compromise and have a salad two out of the seven days. When you are having a salad, also include some root veggies like beets and sweet potatoes. Be a little more liberal with the olive oil and a little more conservative with the vinegar. For the days when you're not eating salads, try to eat cooked foods, which may include soups and stews—especially in the fall and winter months.

4:00PM-4:30 P.M. Teatime! Drink a cup of decaffeinated or herbal tea along with eating some nuts, seeds, or something sweet if you like. Ayurveda suggests avoiding fruit later on in the day, as it can be hard to digest.

7:00-7:30 P.M. For many of us, dinner is the largest meal of the day and, depending when we finish our workday, may be consumed at 8:00 p.m. or later. Digestion has to warm up in the morning, is strong in the middle of the day, and slows down in the evening to allow for anabolic metabolism (the cleaning and replenishing of depleted tissues). Ideally, have a light meal in the evening before 7:30 p.m. This will allow it to be almost fully digested by bedtime at 10:00 p.m.

Recommended Foods for Vata

In my practice, I never say never when it comes to foods, unless of course, they are causing you imbalances. I always suggest moderation when it comes to certain foods and avoidance of foods that may directly increase an already Vatagenic condition. As I've mentioned before, the biggest challenge with those who are predominantly Vata is that they forget to eat and will typically reach for foods that are convenient (salads, packaged goods, and snacks). These foods can be consumed quickly, which often causes bloating and a "heavy" feeling.

Food can make us feel good, heavy, hot, tired, or inflamed. The foods I've listed in this section are generally good for people who are more Vata in nature, or experiencing a Vata imbalance. This is when you get to bring your self-referral powers in—you can make the call as to whether these foods will be right for you at any given time.

Organic, local, and non-GMO foods are always preferred.

GRAINS

It is ideal to eat the following grains as cooked dishes and high-quality breads.

BEST: Amaranth, oats (cooked), quinoa, rice (white or brown), wheat
MODERATION: Barley and millet

AVOID: Buckwheat, corn flour (chips, bread, and tortillas), dry oats (granola), and rye

DAIRY

If you are not following a vegan diet, it's best to use organic and unhomogenized products when available.

BEST: Butter, buttermilk, kefir, whole milk, sour cream, and fresh yogurt

MODERATION: Hard cheeses

AVOID: Ice cream and frozen yogurt (especially in the winter)

SWEETENERS

Moderation is important, as overuse of even the best sweeteners may increase Vata.

BEST: Local and unheated honey, maple syrup, molasses, stevia, and sucanat

AVOID: Brown sugar and white sugar

OILS

Because of the dry quality of Vata, high-quality oils in your diet and on your body are very important to balance Vata.

BEST: Almond, ghee, and sesame

MODERATION: Avocado, coconut, flaxseed, mustard, olive, peanut, and sunflower

AVOID: Safflower oil

FRUITS

Sweet and ripe fruits are best for digestion. Dried fruits are okay in the summertime in high moderation.

BEST: Sweet apples (fresh and baked), apricots, bananas (ripe), black-berries, cantaloupe, cherries, coconut, dates, figs, grapefruit, grapes, lemons, mangoes, nectarines, oranges, papaya, peaches, pears, per-simmons, pineapple, plums, raspberries, strawberries (ripe), and tangerines

MODERATION: Apples (sour) and pomegranate

AVOID: Dried fruits and cranberries

VEGETABLES

Cooked vegetables are generally the best for Vata, as they are easy to digest.

BEST: Avocado, beets, carrots (not as juice), leeks, mustard greens, okra (well cooked), parsnips, shallots, acorn squash, sweet potatoes, and tomatoes (when in season)

MODERATION: Broccoli, cauliflower, celery, corn, cucumber, eggplant, green beans, kale, medium chiles and hot peppers, mushrooms, pota-toes, radishes, seaweed, sweet peas, zucchini, lettuce, spinach and leafy greens (occasional raw use accompanied with a spicy and oily dressing)

AVOID: Alfalfa sprouts, artichokes (unless served with butter and lemon sauce), asparagus, bean sprouts, Brussels sprouts, cabbage (even cooked), onion (especially raw), and snow peas

NUTS AND SEEDS

Raw nuts are best. Have nut butters infrequently and avoid making nuts a central item in your diet.

BEST: Almonds, pumpkin seeds, and sunflower seeds

MODERATION: Cashews, filberts, pecans, pistachios, and sesame seeds

AVOID: Peanuts

MEATS

If you choose to eat meat, consume in a moderate way (3–4 times per week). Favor light animal protein over dark animal protein. Keep your red meat consumption to a minimum. Organic, free-range, and local meats are always preferred.

BEST: Chicken and turkey, duck, freshwater fish

MODERATION: Beef, lamb, pork, seafood, and venison

LEGUMES

Preparing legumes can be challenging because beans need to be soaked overnight to be most digestible. If beans are not prepared properly, you may experience gas and bloating. I've found that sprouted lentils and mung beans are the way to go and are widely available on the internet. Canned beans are okay in moderation.

BEST: Mung beans, chana dal, green lentils, French lentils

MODERATION: Chickpeas (including hummus)

AVOID: Azuki beans, black beans, fava beans, kidney beans, navy beans, and pinto beans

For Vata, food can be moderately spiced and should never be too hot or too bland. Spices help with the digestive process.

BEST: Anise, basil, bay leaf, caraway, cardamom, clove, cumin, dill, fennel, fenugreek, garlic, ginger (fresh), marjoram, mustard, nutmeg, oregano, pepper, peppermint, poppy seeds, rosemary, saffron, sage, spearmint, thyme, and turmeric

MODERATION: Cayenne pepper, cilantro, ginger (dry), horseradish, mustards (very hot), and parsley

AVOID: none

HOW TO BALANCE PITTA

Pitta imbalances occur when there is excess heat, moisture, or an over-consumption of spicy foods or when stressful situations are constant. The first sign of a Pitta imbalance usually presents as loose bowels, diarrhea or hyperacidity, indigestion, and acid reflux. Excess Pitta can also cause fever, night sweats, and occasional headaches or migraines.

Contributing factors to a Pitta imbalance are

* **Excessive stress**
* **Excessive consumption of spicy, oily, and acidic foods (red meat, nightshades, peppers, nuts)**
* **Excessive consumption of alcoholic beverages**
* **Highly competitive routine (always being "on")**
* **Poor sleep hygiene (due to overthinking most situations)**
* **Hot and/or muggy climate**
* **Pitta season (late spring to mid-to-late fall)**

Pitta is the dynamic force in the body that is responsible for transformation and metablolism—not just the ability to transform and metabolize food but also the ability to evaluate and assimilate situations and experiences. It's a well-known fact that people who are predominantly Pitta have often been called out for being too critical or judgmental, but this is the true discerning nature of Pitta, and it is usually expressed in a polite, diplomatic manner. When Pittas go out of balance, however, their diplomacy melts and their searingly critical, deeply judgmental side typically takes the lead.

As Pittas are natural-born leaders, they are warm and inviting and love to work on projects and causes in which "eternal glory" is at stake. Pittas will always start off strong at the beginning of a project—rallying people to their cause and getting their team excited about *their* project. However, when *their* project starts to become monotonous and boring (at least in their mind, which is typically when Pittas need to look at the details of a project), they can quickly lose interest and be on the lookout for the next "glory" project to swing to. This may be because their focus isn't typically on the details of the project but more the adulation that they receive working on a big, bright, and shiny new idea (yes, this is also based on my own experience)!

Pittas prefer to be the big thinkers and the masters of the objective rather than attentive and detail-oriented project managers. This is because Pittas are exceptionally good at big-picture thinking. Words like *visionary*, *rebel*, *revolutionary*, and *trailblazer* generally describe Pittas.

You know you're a Pitta when you send your friends an invitation to a wine tasting and have already texted and called three times to ask them to RSVP even though it's only been eight minutes since you sent out the invite. You answer every call (including the robocalls), are the first to text people back, and email is your life. You like to be constantly connected on as many social media platforms as your mobile device can handle. You don't procrastinate when it comes to communication, which is great; but you do sometimes have a knee-jerk reaction to certain responses, which isn't so great.

Diet and lifestyle recommendations for Pitta aren't about putting out the flames—they're more about understanding the dynamism of the fire and knowing how to use the inferno appropriately, which surprisingly *isn't* all the time! When it comes to balancing yourself through diet and lifestyle edits, remember, you don't have to do it all (even though you might want to, since you know you'll be good at it and you'll be the first to be balanced out of all of your friends—and frenemies). One last note—and because you LOVE taking direction—just a reminder that balance is a marathon, not a sprint. Listen to your heart, not your ego!

Pitta Evening Rituals for Better Sleep

1. After your evening meal, walk 20–30 minutes to help settle your mind.
2. Brush and floss your teeth and scrape your tongue.
3. Get into bed by 10:00 p.m. In the summer months, use lighter covers, perhaps even just a top sheet instead of a comforter.
4. Take ten deep belly breaths to reduce your heart rate and settle your mind and body.

5. If you have difficulty falling asleep, use an ambient noise generator. There are many apps you can download.

6. In the spring and fall, sleep with your windows open slightly. A cooler environment will help you stay asleep if you start having hot flashes (often between midnight and 2:00 a.m.).

7. Lights out by 10:15 p.m.

Pitta Morning Routine for a Productive Day

1. Since you're already awake by 6:00 a.m., get up and spend some of the morning on self-care rather than hitting your email or jumping onto social media.

2. Drink ginger and turmeric tea or hot water with freshly grated ginger before you consume anything else (even though you woke up hungry).

3. Meditate 10–15 minutes and engage in pranayama (breath exercises).

4. If you prefer to exercise in the morning, have a light breakfast (toast, oatmeal) before hitting the gym. Don't forget to plan time to cool down and stretch.

5. Do 20–30 minutes of yoga asana—I recommend a breath-centered Hatha-yoga style (holding poses longer with breath) practice rather than a Vinyasa yoga-style (more flow-oriented) practice.

6. If you have coffee or any other caffeinated beverage, do so after breakfast, and moderate how much caffeine you consume.

7. NOW check your email and social media feeds.

8. Take a warm-to-cool shower, and use soap or body wash designed for your sensitive skin.

9. When you are out of the shower, apply a light and breathable moisturizer with SPF 15 (minimum).

10. Bring your water bottle with you. A copper water bottle is ideal for Pittas, and these are easily purchased on the internet. Alternately, you can use a reusable glass bottle; just make sure you have water with you.

11. Snacks! For Pitta, they're just as important as water, if not more important. Never leave your house without a good selection of snacks. These can be seeds and nuts from the following list or high-quality nutrition bars (in cases of emergency). Fresh is best—do your best!

12. Eat your largest meal at lunch, and when you are eating, don't do it in a place where you'll get aggravated (like in front of your computer or behind the wheel). Remember to chew your food.

13. If you prefer to exercise in the evening, find some time between 6:00 and 7:00 p.m. to do so. For many Pittas, exercise can be a meditation

after a stressful day; just remember to take it easy on your body.

14. Eat a light meal between 7:00 and 7:30 p.m. Again, eat without distraction.

15. Know when to turn off and unplug. There is a reason your mobile device and computer have on/off buttons.

Food and Eating Plan for Pitta

Typically, people who are predominantly Pitta must eat frequently and cannot skip meals, otherwise they get "hangry" (angry because they're hungry). As with many things in a Pitta's day, food consumption can be more like transaction involving calories than about enjoying a good meal. When you are busy and stressed, you may view food consumption as more of a necessity than a time for pleasure; nevertheless, it's important to chew your food properly, as your teeth are in your mouth, not in your stomach. Poorly chewed food can—and invariably will—lead to indigestion and hyperacidity, as will excessive consumption of Pittagenic foods (hot spices, nightshades, alcohol).

Pitta Food Schedule

7:00–7:30 A.M. Enjoy a cooked breakfast, for example, eggs with toasted rice bread or oatmeal with pumpkin seeds. Make sure that you are eating your food mindfully—chewing your food and experiencing the flavors—and not while sitting in front of your computer or behind the wheel, going 80 mph! If you drink coffee or caffeinated teas, eat breakfast before you caffeinate—it will prevent that burning sensation in your belly.

10:00–10:30 A.M. SNACK! It doesn't have to be large, as lunch is just around the corner; so perhaps some seeds and nuts from the following list or a bran muffin. Just make sure that you DON'T wait until noon to eat if you feel the slightest hunger pang.

NOON–1:00 P.M. Showtime! I mean lunchtime! If you can help it, and you probably can if you attempt it, don't schedule any meetings between noon and 1:00 p.m., unless it's a lunch meeting and you are actually eating. Next, enjoy your largest meal now. It will sustain you until at least 4:00 p.m. and allow you to stay focused through the afternoon.

4:00–4:30 P.M. If you are planning on an evening activity before your next meal, like exercising, meeting friends, or a professional engagement, snack now. It will help get you through to 7:00 p.m., when you can have your evening meal. Not snacking in the afternoon may cause you to be excessively hungry by the time you have dinner, and overeating in the evening can and will lead to heartburn or reflux.

7:00–7:30 P.M. Before you dive into your evening meal, take 2–3 deep breaths and give thanks for your meal. Chew your food mindfully, rather than inhaling it as quickly as you can. Savor the flavors, and if it was cooked for you, appreciate the effort someone took to create your meal. Gratitude is the perfect complement to a good meal. Speaking of complements to a meal, if you do consume alcohol, imbibe with moderation. Taken to excess, it can lead cause a Pitta imbalance; specifically, fever, hyperacidity, and in some cases, increased aggression toward others. Enjoy your beverages . . . responsibly.

Recommended Foods for Pitta

For the Pitta person, knowing when blood sugar is getting low is key and having access to high-quality and Pitta-pacifying foods is very important. Therefore, meal planning is key. Make sure that the foods you are eating aren't causing your body to react with inflammatory results, indigestion, acid reflux, and a "fire in the belly" feeling. When foods cause a reaction, observe how the food was consumed as well as what was consumed. You may find that your intolerance to a food is actually to how you're eating it.

Organic and non-GMO foods are best, and go easy on your taste for spicy and acidic foods.

GRAINS

If you're gluten intolerant or celiac, avoid all grains containing gluten.
BEST: Barley, white basmati rice, millet, oats, white rice, wheat/whole wheat
MODERATION: Brown rice (only in acute Pitta conditions, otherwise can be used often)
AVOID: Buckwheat and corn flour products (chips, bread, and tortillas)

DAIRY

If you are not following a vegan diet, consume dairy products in moderation and choose organic unhomogenized milk products when available.

BEST: Unsalted butter, cottage cheese, fresh mozzarella, burrata, cream cheese, ghee, and whole cow's milk and goat's milk

MODERATION: Hard, unsalted cheeses

AVOID: Buttermilk, salted cheeses, sour cream, kefir, cultured milks, yogurt

SWEETENERS

Typically, sweets can reduce Pitta. However, refined sugars can increase the heat of Pitta.

BEST: Sucanat (dried sugar cane), maple syrup, and domestic rice syrup

MODERATION: Dextrose, fructose, honey, raw sugar

AVOID: Molasses and refined sugars

OILS

Use oils in moderation, especially in the summer. Favor oils with a high smoke point (ghee, sesame) when sautéing and frying.

BEST: Coconut, ghee, and olive oil

MODERATION: Avocado, canola, corn, sesame, and sunflower

AVOID: Almond, castor, flaxseed, peanut, and safflower

FRUITS

Sweet and ripe fruits are best. Dried fruits are also good.

BEST: Apples, avocadoes, bananas (ripe), blackberries, cherries, coconut, cranberries, dates, dried fruits, figs, grapes, lemons, limes, nectarines, pineapples, prunes, raisins, raspberries, strawberries, watermelons and all sweet melons

MODERATION: Apricots, bananas (very ripe only), grapefruit, and oranges

AVOID: All sour fruits of any kind; oranges (mandarin), sour pineapple, sour plums, papaya, olives, tangerines, and all unripe fruits

VEGETABLES

Vegetables are best eaten fresh. Fresh green vegetable juices are typically very good to pacify Pitta. Avoid nightshades out of season.

BEST: Alfalfa sprouts, artichoke, asparagus, bean sprouts, bitter melon, broccoli, Brussels sprouts, cabbage, carrots, cauliflower, celery, cilantro, cress, cucumber, green pepper, kale, leafy greens, lettuce, mushrooms, onion (well-cooked), peas, pumpkin, seaweed, and squash

MODERATION: Avocado, beets, bell peppers, corn, garlic (well-cooked), parsley, spinach, sweet potatoes, yellow and vine-ripened tomatoes

AVOID: Chiles, hot peppers, mustard greens, onion (raw), radish, tomato paste, tomato sauce, and any hot or pungent vegetables

NUTS AND SEEDS

Favor nuts and seeds with a lighter oil quality. Roasted is preferred over raw. Avoid nut butters and salted nuts.

BEST: Coconut, sunflower, and pumpkin seeds

MODERATION: Almonds and sesame seeds

AVOID: Brazil nuts, cashews, filberts, macadamia nuts, pecans, pistachios, peanuts, and any other nut not mentioned

MEAT

If you choose to eat animal protein, limit consumption to three to four times a week.

BEST: Chicken, eggs, fresh fish, and turkey

AVOID: Beef, duck, lamb, pork, shellfish, venison, and other red meat

LEGUMES

Prepare your legumes by soaking them overnight. If you don't have time to soak beans, use sprouted beans where available.

BEST: Lentils, chickpeas, mung beans, split peas, soybeans (soy products), and tofu (if tolerated)

MODERATION: Azuki beans, kidney beans, navy beans, and pinto beans

AVOID: Red and yellow lentils

SPICES

For Pitta, food needs to be mild to moderately spiced and never very hot or bland.

BEST: Cardamom, coconut, coriander, dill, fennel, ginger (fresh), lemon verbena, peppermint, saffron, spearmint, and turmeric

MODERATION: Bay leaf, basil, black pepper, caraway, cinnamon, cumin, ginger (powdered), oregano, rosemary, and thyme

AVOID: Cayenne pepper, cloves, fenugreek, garlic (raw), horseradish, marjoram, mustard seeds, nutmeg, poppy seeds, sage, and star anise

HOW TO BALANCE KAPHA

Kapha imbalances typically occur when there is excess damp and cold, an overconsumption of rich, heavy, and oily foods, an absence of physical activity, and a tendency toward withdrawal from social engagements. The first sign of a Kapha imbalance usually presents as mucus in the stool and stools that are darker in color and that sink.

A Kapha imbalance can also present as excess mucus in the nasal cavities and chest, lethargy, seasonal affective disorder (SAD), and, in extreme cases, depression.

CONTRIBUTING FACTORS TO A KAPHA IMBALANCE ARE

- ❊ Habitually staying up late at night
- ❊ Excessive sleep
- ❊ Excessive consumption of dairy products, sweets and candies, oils, and "comfort" or "convenience" foods
- ❊ Lack of physical exercise
- ❊ Getting stuck in routines and habits
- ❊ Becoming overly attached to relationships
- ❊ Attachment to belongings (hoarding)
- ❊ Being reclusive and withdrawn from friends and society
- ❊ Excessively cold and damp climate
- ❊ Kapha season (late winter to mid-to-late spring)

Kapha is the force in the body responsible for cohesion of joints and ligaments, growth and development of the body, and the protective lining in the mouth, stomach, and between the joints. Kapha helps the immune system stay strong and can protect us and fight disease.

Most people who are predominantly Kapha are people the rest of us call our "rocks." Kaphas are the ones we seek out when we are going through a particularly rough patch or when we need a little advice or guidance. Indeed, Kaphas provide us with a stable base, a shoulder to cry on, and a deeply committed friend and confidant. Kaphas keep our secrets and help us get and stay grounded.

Kaphas are generally the epitome of love. They form deep and strong bonds with those who they are close to, and those bonds are typically very tight. Kaphas are nurturing and supportive of their loved ones and will be the protector when their loved ones are threatened or hurt. Kaphas are the protectors of families, the keepers of memories, and the holders of grudges.

When balanced, Kapha love is unconditional. When out of balance, Kaphas can be a little more focused on conditional love. They can become controlling when they feel that the attention from a loved one is waning. Remember, they know your secrets. Extreme Kapha imbalances can lead to hoarding and chronic obesity.

You know you are Kapha if you save all your texts and emails (and some voicemails as well). You are somewhat active on social media but like to observe what's happening in your circle more than interacting with it. When it comes to responding to certain people, you craft caring and considerate notes. When it comes to communicating with people you aren't so keen on, you tend to procrastinate. If that person you're not keen on happens to be a Pitta, you tend drag responding out for as long as you can or at least until your email, text, and voicemail have been completely blown up or melted down by Pitta's persistence.

KAPHA EVENING RITUALS FOR BETTER SLEEP

1. After a light evening meal, walk 20–30 minutes to help stimulate digestion. Avoid alcohol consumption and deserts and sweets.

2. Drink an eight-ounce cup of ginger tea about an hour before bed.

3. Brush and floss your teeth and scrape your tongue.

4. Wash your face.

5. Use a dehumidifier at night if you live in cold and/or damp environment.

6. If you suffer from seasonal allergies, keep your bedroom window closed to avoid excess mucus production.

7. Get into bed by 10:00 p.m. and have your lights out by 10:15 p.m.

KAPHA MORNING ROUTINE FOR A PRODUCTIVE DAY

1. Wake up and get up when you hear your alarm go off at 6:00 a.m. even though you're comfy and it's taken you all night to make your bed this cozy. You're allowed ONE hit to the snooze button only.

2. Once you've peeled yourself from your bed, drink a cup of hot water with fresh ginger or black pepper (or both).

3. Go for an invigorating walk, hike, or active yoga class for at least forty minutes. Remember, it takes a while for you to warm up, but once you're warm, you can keep going.

4. Set your intention for the day. It can be something you want to accomplish at work or home. You can write your intention on a small piece of paper and keep it with you at your desk. Keep it positive and uplifting, and revisit it throughout the day.

5. Dry-brush before showering. Dry brushing not only brings circulation back to the skin, it also helps to drain the lymphatic system, stimulate digestion, and reduce ama. To dry-brush, start with a soft, natural bristle brush. Making circular motions, start with your feet, and work your way up your legs, stomach, arms, and back—avoid the heart. This process can take 8–10 minutes.

6. **Oil pulling.** As part of your oral health ritual, use 1–2 tablespoons of organic sesame oil, and swish it around your mouth for 15–20 minutes. Oil pulling can help reduce ama in your digestive system and improve digestion. If you're feeling extra industrious, you can oil pull as you're dry brushing! Spit the oil/saliva mix into into a paper cup or trash bag and cover it with a napkin or paper towel to absorb the oil.

7. Take a warm to hot shower but not scalding hot. The heat will help stimulate circulation and break up excess oil in the skin.

8. Use an invigorating soap or body wash containing rosemary, mint, or tea tree oil.

9. Dress in clothes that inspire confidence in you and keep you feeling light.

10. Eat a hot and light breakfast if you're hungry—perhaps oatmeal with a little bit of honey and cinnamon or some fresh fruit from the list of recommended foods.

11. Sip hot water throughout the day. You can bring boiled water in a thermos and sip a cup every thirty minutes or so. Hot water helps to stimulate metabolism, removes ama and waste from your digestive system, and promotes weight management. Boil your water on a stove, not in a microwave.

12. If you have a sedentary job, get up and move for five minutes every hour. This can be a simple stand-and-stretch at your desk.

13. Eat your largest meal between noon and 1:00 p.m., and eat heavy foods in moderation. Favor cooked meals that are lighter in oils and salt. You can even make your own spice mix to bring with you to make the flavor of your meal more exciting.

14. If you start to feel sleepy between 2:00 p.m. and 4:00 p.m., avoid a trip to the vending machine or coffee shop. Have a cup of ginger tea and walk around your office for 5–10 minutes to stimulate circulation and increase your oxygen intake.

15. Eat a light meal between 6:30 p.m. and 7:00 p.m. if you're hungry.

16. Avoid binge-watching TV shows. This may cause you to stay up until the late hours of the night, which in turn will cause you to sleep past your alarm.

Food and Eating Plan for Kapha

People who are predominantly Kapha in nature typically experience a low-grade hunger most of the day. Unlike their Vata and Pitta counterparts who can eat up to five times a day, it's recommended in

Ayurveda that Kaphas eat three to four times per day—still enjoying the largest meal at lunch and having lighter meals for breakfast and dinner.

If you are craving something sweet, be mindful of the amount. Rather than eating the entire bar of chocolate, maybe savor just one square. Excessive consumption of Kaphagenic foods (dairy, sweets, simple carbohydrates) will cause lethargy, excess mucus production, sluggish digestion, and weight gain.

Kapha Food Schedule

7:00-7:30 A.M. If you are hungry, enjoy a hot breakfast of rice and vegetables if you prefer a savory meal or oatmeal with cinnamon and a little local honey. If you aren't hungry, start with a cup of ginger tea and bring some fresh fruit with you to work. You may feel hungry a little later in the morning, and fresh fruit is typically better for your Kapha constitution than a candy bar.

NOON-1:00 P.M. If you are eating lunch at a restaurant within walking distance of your work, walk, don't drive. Even though this is your largest meal of the day, avoid the tendency to order a sandwich with French fries and extra ketchup. Instead, choose foods that are cooked with less oil and provide some fiber. Soup and a salad are good options, but don't drown your salad in creamy dressing. If you are bringing your lunch to work, be mindful of eating it away from your desk. Perhaps eat your lunch with a coworker outside so that you can take a short walk after lunch. I know this is challenging, as you can dive into your work and tend to be a little antisocial, but the companionship will help you stay light and buoyant.

6:30-7:00 P.M. Before you start prepping your evening meal, check in with yourself. If you've had a stressful day, your first inclination may be to hit the snacks as you decide what you're going to make for dinner. Give yourself a few minutes to decompress from your workday before prepping food, and maybe do a short breath exercise or meditation. Choose meals that are easier to prepare with less cooking time, so that you aren't eating late into the evening. Avoid foods high in dairy, heavy starches, and red meat.

Recommended Foods for Kapha

For Kaphas, food can be a double-edged sword: On the one hand, it provides necessary sustenance; on the other, it's a stress release and can be addictive. When Kaphas are stressed, they will reach for foods that will essentially "give them a hug" in the form of a big shot of dopamine (the "reward" hormone). It's not that I'm suggesting that Kaphas eat salads for the rest of their lives—what I am suggesting is that understanding your stress patterns, especially where food is concerned, will help you be mindful and manage the amount of Kaphagenic foods you consume when stressed. In this case, mindful eating with minimally processed, organic, and non-GMO foods is best.

GRAINS

Consuming grains in excess typically leads to a deeper Kapha imbalance. Favor grains that are higher in protein.

BEST: Amaranth, barley, basmati rice, buckwheat, corn flour, quinoa, white basmati rice, and oats

MODERATION: Millet and rye

AVOID: Short-grain white and brown rice, wheat

DAIRY

When balancing Kapha, eat only a little dairy, or avoid it altogether. If milk is to be included in your diet, favor unhomogenized milk, and boil the milk to make it easier it digest.

BEST: Goat milk

MODERATION: Ghee

AVOID: Butter, buttermilk, cheese, cream, cottage cheese, ice cream, sour cream, whole milk, and yogurt

SWEETENERS

Excess sweeteners can increase Kapha. Favor natural sugars in moderation.

BEST: Local raw honey

MODERATION: Fructose, maple syrup, and molasses

AVOID: Raw sugar, white sugar, and brown sugar

OILS

Use oils in small amounts only. Even the best oils, if overused, will increase Kapha.

BEST: Canola, corn, flaxseed, mustard, safflower, and sunflower oil

MODERATION: Avocado, coconut, olive, and sesame oil

AVOID: Almond, peanut oil

FRUITS

Fruits that are more astringent in nature are best for Kapha, as excess sugar can increase the water and earth elements.

BEST: Apples, cherries, cranberries, grapefruit, pomegranate, prunes, and raisins

MODERATION: Apricots, lemon, lime, papaya, and pineapple

AVOID: Avocado, bananas, berries (raspberries, blackberries, blueberries, strawberries), cantaloupe, coconut, dates, figs, grapes, mango, melons, oranges, peaches, pears, persimmons, plums, tangerines, and watermelons

VEGETABLES

Vegetable can be consumed cooked in the fall and winter and raw (in salads) in the spring and summer.

BEST: Alfalfa sprouts, artichoke, asparagus, bell peppers, broccoli, Brussels sprouts, cabbage, cauliflower, celery, cilantro, chiles, corn, green beans, kale, hot peppers, leafy greens, lettuce, mushrooms, onions, potatoes, radish, rutabagas, spinach, turnips, pumpkin, seaweed, and squashes

MODERATION: Mushrooms and tomatoes

AVOID: Beets, cucumber, eggplant, okra, sweet potatoes, water chestnuts, zucchini, and all squash

NUTS AND SEEDS

Because of their oily qualities seeds are preferred over nuts for Kapha. If sprouted nuts (almonds, cashews, and so on) are available, moderate consumption is appropriate for Kapha.

BEST: Sunflower and pumpkin seeds

MODERATION: Sesame seeds

AVOID: Almonds, Brazil nuts, cashews, coconuts, filberts, lotus seeds, macadamia nuts, pecans, pistachios, peanuts, and walnuts

MEATS

If you choose to eat meat, limit consumption to two to three times a week.

BEST: Chicken and turkey (dark meat only), fish, and rabbit

MODERATION: Eggs

AVOID: Beef, duck, lamb, pork, shellfish, and venison

LEGUMES

Legumes must be properly processed prior to consumption. Soak legumes overnight and rinse them prior to cooking to avoid excess gas.

BEST: Dal, mung beans, green lentils, and split peas

MODERATION: Azuki beans, black beans, fava beans, kidney beans, lima beans, and pinto beans

AVOID: Black lentils and chickpeas

SPICES

Spices that are pungent (turmeric) and astringent (basil) and are good for digestion (ginger and black pepper) are preferred. When using salt, favor pink Himalayan salt, and use sparingly.

BEST: Basil, black pepper, chamomile, caraway, cardamom, cinnamon, cloves, coriander, cumin, dill, fennel, fenugreek, garlic, ginger, horseradish, hyssop, marjoram, mustard, nutmeg, oregano, peppermint, poppy seeds, rosemary, saffron, sage, spearmint, star anise, thyme, turmeric, and any other hot spices not mentioned

MODERATION: Cayenne pepper

AVOID: Salt

CONCLUSION

Starting on your own path to balanced health is not easy—especially with so much information available. The journey on the path to balanced health is the destination, and we have to approach our journey at our own pace in order for it to be sustainable. As Ayurveda provides us with somewhat of a user's manual to operate our doshas, following even just the simpler guidelines about diet and lifestyle for your body type will help prevent an imbalance or illness from occurring.

My recommendation to my clients on this is to always follow the 80/20 rule: 80 percent of the time you're eating for your body type and reducing your stress with yoga, exercise, or meditation; and the other 20 percent of the time, you're throwing caution to the wind by staying up past your bedtime and eating foods that aren't always the best choice—and not beating yourself up for it. Ayurvedic medicine isn't an all-or-nothing system; it accounts for those times when you're unable to always follow the "correct" path. When you start to go out of balance, your body will send out simple reminders when it's time to get back on the path.

I hope this book has inspired you to start or restart your journey to balanced health. I would like to offer you these words of encouragement: *Intention*, *attention*, and *direction*. Find and set your intention for your health goals. This may be getting better sleep, clearer skin, or better digestion. With your intention set, keep focusing your attention on your journey. Know that even if you fall off the path, you can always get back on it. You have the knowledge and self-referral to do so. Keep your direction, and know that as you start reaching your health goals, be prepared to evolve your attention.

Lastly, be patient with yourself. Bodies don't go out of balance overnight, so it's only natural to need to spend the time to help bring yours back to balance.

ENDNOTES

1   Narayanaswamy, V., "Origin and Development of Ayurveda," https://www.ncbi.nlm.nih.gov/pmc/articles/PMC3336651/pdf/ASL-1-1.pdf (April 17, 2019).

2   Ibid.

3   "Ayurvedic Medicine: In Depth," National Center for Complementary and Integrative Health, https://nccih.nih.gov/health/ayurveda/introduction.htm (April 17, 2019).

4   "Vacation Pay," Workplace Fairness, https://www.workplacefairness.org/vacation-pay (April 17, 2019).

5   "Healthy Lifestyle: Stress Management," Mayo Clinic, https://www.mayoclinic.org/healthy-lifestyle/stress-management/in-depth/stress-symptoms/art-20050987 (April 17, 2019).

6   "Holiday entitlements," NIDirect, https://www.nidirect.gov.uk/articles/holiday-entitlements (April 17, 2019).

7   "Complementary and Alternative Healthcare: Is it Evidence-Based?" International Journal of Health Sciences, https://www.ncbi.nlm.nih.gov/pmc/articles/PMC3068720/ (April 17, 2019).

8   "The Functional Medicine Approach," The Institute for Functional Medicine, https://www.ifm.org/functional-medicine/what-is-functional-medicine/ (April 17, 2019).

9   "Health and Economic Costs of Chronic Diseases," CDC, https://www.cdc.gov/chronicdisease/about/costs/index.htm (April 17, 2019).

10   Benjamin, R., "The National Prevention Strategy," https://www.ncbi.nlm.nih.gov/pmc/articles/PMC3185312/ (April 17, 2019).

ACKNOWLEDGMENTS

My journey started with Virginia Treherne-Thomas, who introduced me to Ayurveda and yoga in 1988 on one of her trips to Maharishi Mahesh Yogi's clinic in Lancaster, Massachusetts, and Kripalu in Lenox, Massachusetts. It's with deep gratitude that you introduced me to this path.

Thank you to my mentors, Dr. Robert Keith Wallace and the Wallace family, Dr. Stuart Rothenberg, Dr. Nancy Lonsdorf, and Dr. Hemant Gupta, for guiding and encouraging me in my career in Ayurveda.

Thank you to my team and community at Well Sonoma for believing in my vision for integrative health.

Much love to Arek Reeder, Devi Norton, and Peggy Foley for being part of so much of my journey.

Thank you to Sam Treherne-Thomas and to my husband, Jim Kuhner, and the Kuhner family for adopting me as one of your own.

Finally, a big thank-you to Kate Zimmermann, who guided me through the process of writing this book.

ABOUT THE AUTHOR

Chronic illness and obesity led Deacon at the age of sixteen to a fateful meeting with a local Ayurvedic doctor, and that meeting created a seismic shift in his perception of nutrition, health, and physical balance. Heeding the advice of his doctor, Deacon was empowered to understand what was causing him to be sick; and the steps to reclaiming his health were clear and simple. Deacon modified his diet, started to practice yoga, and shed more than 140 pounds.

Deacon's interest in Ayurvedic studies continued at Maharishi University of Management in Fairfield, Iowa, where he deepened his knowledge and decided that it was his calling to become an Ayurvedic clinician.

However, it was during his sixteen-year career working in the trenches of global advertising and branding that he was able to hone his communication skills, thus enabling him to convey the complex ideas and concepts of Ayurveda and yoga in a comprehensive and practical manner.

Deacon continues to teach his practical approach to Ayurveda and yoga at Maharishi University of Management, where he has been a guest faculty member, adjunct professor, and co-creator of their M.S. program in Maharishi Ayurveda and integrative medicine.

Deacon is the owner of Well Sonoma, an integrative medical clinic focusing on personalized medicine through Ayurveda, yoga, and other complementary modalities, in Santa Rosa, California.

INDEX